Praise for the Author

My injury required two major spinal operations both of which were a failure and resulted in a loss of quality in my life – poor mobility and unable to drive my car for two years. All my doctors told me they could do no more for me, unbearable pain and numerous drugs. I feel fantastic after a number of treatments with Suzanne. My mobility has improved out of this world. My pain has almost gone and I am able to play with my grandchildren. Today I feel a genuine 90–95% improvement within my body and I would highly recommend Suzanne.

Richard T.

Diagnosed osteoporosis with pain 24/7 for the past 15 weeks. My working career was over, so my doctor said. Pain level was more than 10 out of 10. Had to use walking stick and a wheel chair. Constant pain – morphine did little to shift. Quality of life since treatment with Suzanne, out of this world! Pain level after treatment minus 1 out of 10. Best thing ever!

Max E.

I had a prolapsed disc on the right-hand side of my back at L4/5 with L5 root compression (as per X-ray). I hurt my back doing a simple chore under the house and the pain went down the side of my bottom, down the outside of my knee towards my ankle. I had been unable to get any sleep, had tried hot packs, pain killers, etc. I was sent to a specialist to receive treatment but on examination of the x-rays he stated that no surgery was needed and suggested physiotherapy. I attended Suzanne's Clinic instead and after three or four treatments I received relief from the severe pain I was suffering.

Thelma G.

I've had five major abdominal surgeries, the first at age five to remove a ten-pound fluid cyst from my abdomen. As a consequence, my core is very weak and from time to time my lower back becomes extremely painful and I suffer from debilitating sciatic pain and muscle spasm. Suzanne is the only therapist that has ever been able to relieve the pain and get me moving freely again. I am also a chronic asthmatic whose first breath, according to my mother, was a wheeze. My ability to breathe and breathe deeply is greatly enhanced following a treatment from Suzanne who has a unique gift.

Karen M.

After spending 14 years in the military with deployments to East Timor and Afghanistan, I have a lot of tension in my body. The physical wear and tear requires weekly maintenance and I've used several bodywork methods over the years. Chiro, physio, massage and osteo have all offered limited relief. After receiving Bowen with Suzanne, I was able to turn my head in both directions without pain for the first time in years. The techniques she used on my upper back enabled me to take full breaths without pain or restriction. Since leaving the military, I've been teaching yoga and find it helps with chronic stress, past trauma and physical injuries. Bowen helps to further open the body, reducing pain and relieving tension. It's a perfect complement to a physical practice and enhances the benefits of yoga.

Chris T-L., Frontline Yoga.

From small, niggling, consistent pains to excruciating back pain I have had extremely positive results with Suzanne. The pain relief has been quickly noticeable from the time of the treatment. I especially like that treatment is only necessary to deal with a problem for a small number of sessions (usually two or three) as opposed to a never-ending and expensive regime offered by alternative treatment fields. I have no hesitation in recommending for a range of ailments and have done so on many occasions to family, friends and acquaintances.

Terri W.

Over the years my back and neck would have a tendency to seize up leaving me in considerable pain and discomfort. The only relief I found was after treatment with Suzanne and within 48 hours I was as good as new.

Gayle S.

After living with joint aches and pains in my hips, all through my legs as well as tension and stress in my upper back and shoulders, I began working with Suzanne to realign my back and bring back balance to firstly my spine which in turn released the tension and stresses held within my muscles. The sessions were very relaxing, gave pain relief and I slept much better afterwards. Suzanne's knowledge and her gentle approach to the healing of the body is extensive. I was amazed at how non-invasive the procedure is and the direct positive effect it has on the body. Suzanne's patience, sincerity, listening and understanding of what is needed to heal the body at different times in my life has been genuine.

Janelle C.

I had arthritis in my back and it affected my walking. Had it for months, and after going to physiotherapy for many months and no improvements, was recommended therapy with Suzanne. My condition has improved greatly. Lately had a pinched nerve in the neck and after treatment that has greatly improved, much, much better.

Win F.

I had some Bowen Therapy done two years ago now with Suzanne and had three sessions. I have no more back pain and so I'm pain free. Previous to the treatment I had pain for two years. Everyday sciatic pain down to the toes, had trouble sitting and standing. I found it just brilliant.

Ian J.

I had basic back pain in 2004 which eventually resulted in a left hip replacement in 2005. This was unsuccessful and further operations were required in 2009 and 2010. Pain in the hip area continued. In 2016, I was diagnosed with curvature of the spine (scoliosis) and osteoporosis of the spine – severe. In November 2016 I was placed in hospital rehabilitation, much of the treatment in rehab involved physio. In the past I have received much relief from Suzanne and Bowen Therapy and my doctor has suggested this treatment would be less invasive. I find that I have much relief and my quality of life is improving with this treatment from Suzanne. I am over 70 years of age and it also helps me breathe better.

Margaret B.

After my son injured his ankle at sport, we turned to Bowen Therapy for help. I am so grateful to Suzanne for her gentle releases, which reduced the muscle tightness in my son's legs. The sessions have improved his range of motion greatly and he is now running freely, without any pain. He looks forward to sessions.

Petrea C.

I began seeing Suzanne 14 years ago after injuring my lower back. I spent two years in constant agony going from chiropractic, physiotherapy, etc., anything I could find for relief. Nothing. Pains from lower back to feet, no feeling in my toes. Cried constantly until one day a man suggested Suzanne to my husband, what a lifesaver she has been for me. I must stress not an immediate miracle but with her reassurance and confidence and my husband's, I persisted. What did I have to lose, I was desperate. Took twelve months to come good and I will never let anyone else treat me again with any other treatment but Bowen! So gentle but my goodness so effective. A beautiful therapist and incredible treatment has given me quality of life back. Thank you from the bottom of my heart.

Jenny M.

Back pain, neck and shoulder tightness have been problems that I have dealt with for many years. After having foot surgery, my gait has changed, thus my posture has changed. Suzanne assessed me then explained how she could help. My experience has been amazing. Suzanne's clear voice and gentleness relaxes you and the session is enjoyable and so helpful. I look forward to my next session. I am convinced that it works and has made a difference for me. Suzanne is knowledgeable and caring and I am grateful for the support and relief she has given me.

Pauline M.

DRUG FREE
PAIN RELIEF

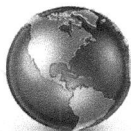

GLOBAL
PUBLISHING
G R O U P

Global Publishing Group
Australia • New Zealand • Singapore • America • London

DRUG FREE PAIN RELIEF

The TRUTH About How to Avoid Pain Even if You've Tried Other Methods!

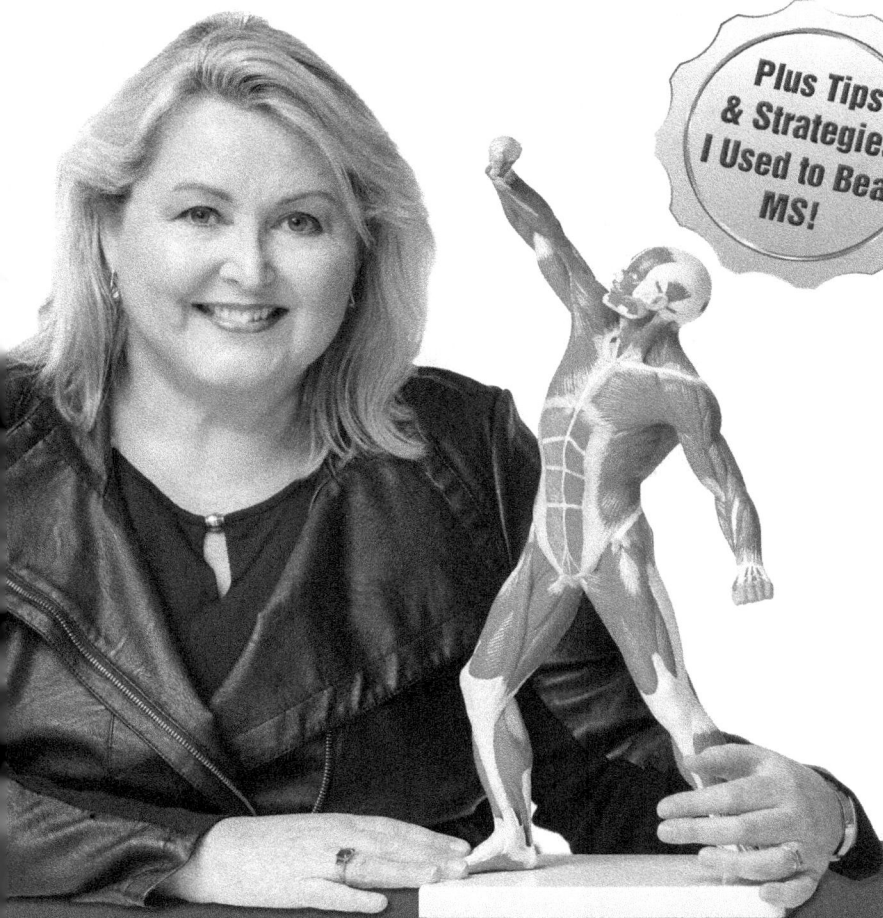

Plus Tips & Strategies I Used to Beat MS!

SUZANNE McTIER-BROWNE

BA, GDM, MBA, Advanced Bowen Therapist, Reflexologist & Massage Therapist

DISCLAIMER

All the information, techniques, skills and concepts contained within this publication are of the nature of general comment only and are not in any way recommended as individual advice. The intent is to offer a variety of information to provide a wider range of choices now and in the future, recognising that we all have widely diverse circumstances and viewpoints. Should any reader choose to make use of the information contained herein, this is their decision, and the contributors (and their companies), authors and publishers do not assume any responsibilities whatsoever under any condition or circumstances. It is recommended that the reader obtain their own independent advice.

First Edition 2017

Copyright © 2017 Suzanne McTier-Browne

A catalogue record for this book is available from the National Library of Australia

Published by Global Publishing Group
PO Box 517 Mt Evelyn, Victoria 3796 Australia
Email info@GlobalPublishingGroup.com.au

For further information about orders:
Phone: +61 3 9726 4133 or Fax +61 3 8648 6871

I dedicate this book to you, my new friend, battling pain (or maybe you've been there, done that and never want to go there again).

You are not powerless and you are not alone. I have faith that you have the strength to transform and set yourself free. You are a pain relief warrior!

My sincere hope is that you love yourself enough to make this sacred commitment.

Best wishes always!

Suzanne McTier-Browne

EXTRA BONUS

I can't give you everything
you need to know about drug free
pain relief in one small book.

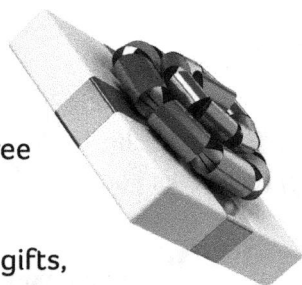

So I've created some extra special gifts,
just for you. You'll find lots of pain relief
bonuses that will help fast track
your success.

There are tools and resources to help
strengthen your body and mind
so that you can become
pain free.

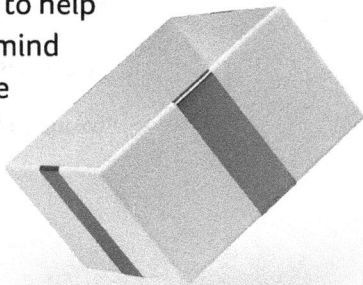

**To claim your FREE BONUS OFFERS and
success tools, go to:**

www.DrugFreePainReliefBook.com

Acknowledgements

Wow, where to begin? Firstly to the two gentlemen who blessed my life but who were both taken away tragically before their time. My father Malcolm was a charismatic, charitable and highly intelligent man. My husband Steven also had the ability to befriend and charm people with his honesty and love for life. I have been so lucky to have had two wonderful men truly love and believe in me.

A big thank you to the beautiful women in my family. My daughters Cassandra and Mikaela are my inspiration. It breaks my heart that you also lost your father at such young ages but I am in awe at how clever, kind and capable you both are – truly shining stars. My mother Kathleen, who when my father passed, picked herself up and started a successful business while providing loving support to my brother and I. Thank you to my brother Gregory, a gentle giant who is always there for me and his loving family, Karen, Hannah, Jackson and Thomas (in heaven). Thanks also to my father-in-law, Desmond Browne.

Sincere thank you to George Hardy who at a very dark time in my life helped save me through his bodywork skills. Also thanks go to the late Lady Cilento whose books on nutrition, vitamins and minerals provided me with powerful information to support and heal my body.

Heartfelt gratitude to the master of body structural correction and gentle pain relief, the late Thomas Bowen. His amazing Bowen Technique treats the body in such a respectful and clever way. Sincere thanks to Oswald & Elaine Rentsch for documenting and teaching Mr Bowen's work and to my other instructors – Robyn Wood, Desley Faulks, Gael Cox, Anne Schubert and Margaret Spicer.

In my thirst for further knowledge I also trained in other valuable therapies and techniques and so thank Heather Edwards and Catherine Lee (Reflexology); Jenny Lee (Baby Reflexology); Linda Williams (Hot Stone Reflexology); Ross Emmett (Emmett Technique); Lisa Black and Col Murray (ISBT); Vincent Leo (Remedial Massage); D. Gary Young,

Dr David Stewart, Artemis, Cliff Winkleman and Riga Walsh (Raindrops & Vitaflex Technique); Eugene Piccinotti (Thought Field Therapy) and Colleen Keetley (ENAR Therapy System). Thanks to fellow therapists Jenny Healy, Christine Hayman, Judy Smoothy, Veronica Germann, Fiona Davis, Dee Kynoch, Matilda Smith and Bill Mather.

A big thank you to Dr Jo Turner who invited me early in my therapist career to join her at the Family Medical Practice. So grateful for the years I worked there with all the wonderful doctors and staff (also at the second Family Medical Practice).

So much respect for Young Living Essential Oils and the work of D. Gary Young. Having visited several Young Living farming operations, I am in awe of the expertise and quality. Also thankful for my Young Living family and friends (Artemis, Neena Love, Fiona Cookson, Natalie Giles, Aj Ley, Bill and Carla Green and the rest of you so important but too numerous to mention individually).

My dear friends who provided moral support and valuable feedback – Gayle and Rod Shannen, Kaylene Paradine (also my stretch and exercise photographer) and Janelle Cooke. Thanks also to my health and fitness models Mikaela and Cassandra McTier-Browne. Gratitude to my publisher, Darren and Jacqui Stephens and their wonderful team, including my book manager, Kelly Mayne.

Over the years I have also been inspired by giants in their fields such as the Dalai Lama, Deepak Chopra, Oprah Winfrey, Dr John Gray, Dr Mehmet C Oz, Dr Joseph Mercola, Dr Phil McGraw, Louise Hay, Tony Robbins, Sir Richard Branson, Darren Hardy, Dr Wayne Dyer, Rhonda Byrne, Bear Grylls and Dwayne The Rock Johnson.

And finally, I am indebted to the thousands of clients who have invited me into their lives. Thank you to those who provided testimonials and also those who spread the word personally to others in need. Working at the Good Health & Pain Relief Clinic, has given me such joy and a real purpose for which I am so grateful.

Contents

Introduction

Most of us have either experienced pain personally or know someone dealing with pain. Chronic pain affects one in five Australians, including children, and one in three people over 65. Back pain, arthritis and musculoskeletal conditions are the most common causes and account for 40% of early retirement from the workforce. According to Painaustralia, by 2050 and as Australia's population ages, an estimated five million people will be struggling to deal with their chronic pain.

Of course, dealing with pain is not just an Australian problem, it is a global epidemic. The American Academy of Pain Medicine advises that chronic pain affects more than 100 million Americans and more than 1.5 billion people worldwide. It costs the American health care system approximately $300 billion annually while at least another $300 billion is additionally lost due to decreased productivity.

So the costs are financial as well as personal which can add even further to pain and stress. In an effort to deal with this physical and often emotional pain, prescription pain killers can sometimes be misused or abused. Used in the right situation they are powerful and life-saving but as a long term pain strategy there can sometimes be complications. In a review of opioid-related mortality in the United States and Canada, Dr Nicholas King and colleagues from the Biomedical Ethics Unit and the Department of Epidemiology, Biostatistics and Occupational Health, McGill University, found:

> *Deaths involving prescription opioid analgesics, including hydrocodone, oxycodone, hydromorphone, and methadone, have surpassed deaths from heroin and cocaine combined. In 2010, the 11th consecutive year in which drug overdose deaths increased, 75% of all pharmaceutical overdose deaths involved opioids, and prescription opioids were involved in 16,651 deaths in the United States.*

Unfortunately USA and Canada are not alone with those sobering statistics – a 2017 ABC News article states that in Australia, 800 people a year die from prescription drug overdoses which include commonly prescribed opioids such as oxycontin, fentanyl, codeine and morphine.

But enough of statistics. Those of us who have been in pain or those who are currently battling pain conditions already know the personal and emotional costs. From experience I also know that when you are in excruciating pain, you haven't the energy, mental clarity or care factor to read through thousands of words detailing definitions of pain, anatomy diagrams etc., you just want to get to the part about how to deal with it. If you are in that urgent situation, you might like skip the rest of this introduction and start at Chapter Two.

So here is what this book is not. It is not an academic book or anatomy text detailing the complexities and theories of pain. This book is also not an instruction manual to teach the therapies I use and recommend. My goal is not to teach you body science but to give you information about the strategies that worked for me and my clients and to provide practical tools and techniques that you can use to help turn your life around and live pain free!

Also please note, I'm not anti-pharmaceutical or anti-pain medications. There are some great pain and life-saving medications. If they are working for you – thank goodness for them! It's just that prescribed pain medications did not work for me in the past and so I had to ascertain the cause of my pain and then work to eliminate it at the source.

For the vast majority of people I come into contact in a clinic situation, pain medications are also not working for them and so many have been left in painful limbo. Sometimes those medications may have worked well initially but because the cause of the pain was not addressed, they lost their potency and good effect. Sometimes the side effects outweigh the benefits.

While pain meds are invaluable to handle pain in acute or emergency situations, for long-term chronic pain they can sometimes be temporary 'band-aid' solutions that may come with side effects and decreases in efficiency. So if you do not want to be reliant on prescription medications forever, again it becomes important to deal with WHY you are getting pain and HOW you are going to fix it for the long term.

Of course everybody is different, medications and treatments that have worked for others with similar conditions cannot always be guaranteed to work for you. Different genetics, raised in diverse environments, having been exposed to unique combinations of chemicals and toxins, eating differently, having various personalities, emotional states and abilities to handle stress and disease etc. Likewise the therapies and techniques that worked for me and for my clients cannot be guaranteed but at least they are safe to try and will support your health in other ways.

The reality is that no one can give you a guarantee because people are wonderful, complex beings who can be massively unpredictable. Sometimes the only way to know whether something will work for you is to try, and if that doesn't work try something else. Keep taking positive action and don't get angry if your doctor, therapist, medication or supplement doesn't work straight away for you. More time might be needed, maybe some fine-tuning or perhaps it's not the right answer for you just now.

I know it can be hard (sometimes excruciatingly hard) but be grateful that you are learning along the way and it is important to keep moving forward. Take responsibility and realise that you have to do something different if you want different and positive results. If you become complacent and keep doing what you have always done, then chances are that you will keep getting the same results and the same pain!

When I was diagnosed with MS and orthodox medicine had no cure and no hope for me, I had to be determined (some called it stubborn) and try out things for myself and persist, keep going even when there was no hope. If I'd given up and prepared for my demise like my neurologist had advised me all those years ago, I would never have recovered, got married, had children, have a wonderful career helping people or be here writing this book. So if you are currently in a similar situation, my heart goes out to you but please whatever you do, don't give up.

Patience and commitment are extremely important as usually the longer you've had a pain condition, the more time and effort it takes to turn it around. It's a bit like the momentum of a runaway train. Once pain has become entrenched, it develops a momentum of its own which requires a lot of effort to firstly slow down the progression and then to gradually bring it to a stop. It then takes another mighty effort to reverse the direction of that "pain train" and commence your healing journey. So be prepared to put in your best effort – this is the most important work you'll ever do!

> *"Turn around that pain train, you are the driver and in control of your journey to a pain free and happy life!"*
>
> **Suzanne McTier-Browne**

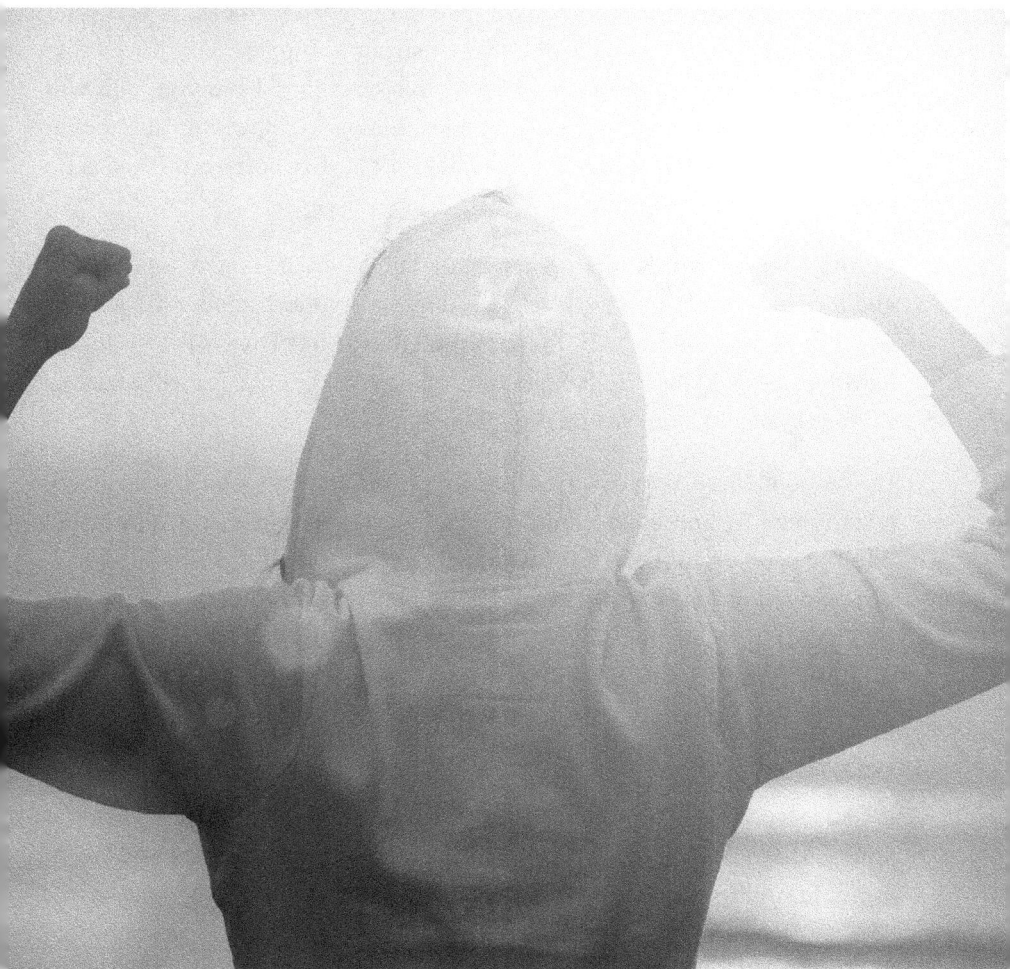

CHAPTER 1

How I Beat MS!

CHAPTER 1

How I Beat MS!

I was only 22 when I was given a death sentence. My neurologist had just got back the results from my brain scans, eyesight and hearing tests.

"You have MS, multiple sclerosis. You are in the typical age-group and your symptoms are also typical. Your MS is progressing very rapidly, I estimate that you have less than a year. So go home and get your affairs in order, I seriously doubt you will reach your 23rd birthday. If you want to do something or go on a small trip – I strongly suggest do it now while you still have a bit of mobility. I know that next time I see you, you will be in a wheelchair and once that happens, things will speed up and then it will just be a matter of months … well that's it. I'm sorry but there is no treatment for multiple sclerosis."

I remember his words like it was yesterday. My neurologist was sincere and looking deeply into my eyes to see if I was understanding the gravity of what he was saying. Of course I understood but I was still finding it hard to digest. I was numb, somehow I just couldn't accept what he was saying. It was like he was talking about someone else.

How could there be no way of treating this? I was young, previously healthy and fit and even though I was in excruciating pain I didn't feel like I was going to die. I felt so sorry for my mother, I didn't want her to lose a loved one so soon after my father's passing. I remember looking at my neurologist and thinking – really, is that it? Why are you giving up on me? Surely there is something we can do? We just could not lose another member of my family. My mother sat silently beside me holding my hand tightly.

It had only been ten months since my father's passing. He died at the young age of 51, in part due to medical error, so it had been a huge shock to my family to suddenly lose such a loving family man.

So yes, I did totally understand what my neurologist was saying about my condition but whether I was going to accept it, was another thing, I was determined to get better. Maybe it was my Scottish ancestry that brought out the fighter in me but there was no way I was giving up or leaving my mother and brother to grieve another family loss.

But I also knew I was in real trouble and I had to move fast. My deterioration had started just a couple of months previously when at first I thought I was just being clumsy. Over the next few weeks I began dropping things, predominately with my left hand, and then alarmingly also with my right. Even light objects such as a pen or cup would fall from my grasp.

Then came the walking into walls and misjudging corners, I always had bruises. I was unable to walk in a straight line no matter how I tried and always veered off to the left. But somehow that didn't really worry me until the lightning and fireworks.

I began seeing flashes of fierce bright light in my vision which quickly escalated and soon I had a whole light show going on – lightning and fireworks continually firing. It got so bad I would even see it when I closed my eyes. Trying to sleep at night was frightening and frustrating with light exploding and popping until I eventually fell asleep but it was there again first thing in the morning once I awoke, even before I opened my eyes. I thought my brain was somehow short-circuiting.

Then came the tightening of my joints and being unable to move freely, I progressively slowed down and stiffened. At the time, I had really been enjoying life. I had a great job, I'd finished the hard work and stress of university study, I had a wonderful boyfriend Steven (who later became my husband) and I loved physical exercise.

Even though I owned a car, I would ride my bike to the local tennis court complex to swim in the pool and workout in the weights room (this was in the days before trendy gyms). I also liked to do a bit of jogging but as I started to become clumsy, I also became really, really tired. I began to worry about falling off my bike and so gradually had to stop all the activity I previously enjoyed.

I was hurting all over. It was excruciating to walk up stairs and as we lived in a double-storey house, I often crawled up on my hands and knees. It hurt to walk down stairs and because of my pain and clumsiness, I would normally sit on my bottom and slide awkwardly down each step. Alarmingly quickly for a previously healthy and energetic 22 year old, I was slowing down, getting stiff, sore, weak and clumsy. And still it kept on progressing.

My mother and I left the neurologist, totally numb. I was given an appointment to see him again in three months along with information about getting a wheelchair. The following weeks passed in a haze of disbelief as I researched everything I could about MS and natural ways to heal the body.

Because of the intense pain I was in, my aunt suggested a session with her therapist in Murwillumbah, northern NSW – George Hardy, who had helped her get relief from back ache. Mum and I decided to travel down to see George immediately (though in those days it took around 14 hours to drive by car).

On my first visit, George took one look at me and shook his head. He later told my mother that my body was so structurally misaligned, he could tell I had been in a really bad accident in my past. And he was right!

When I was 13, in my first year of high school, I was hit by a car. I had ridden my bicycle to my friend's place during a school lunch break and was waiting for her, across the road from her house which was on the down side of a small hill. The narrow centre of the road was bitumen but the sides or shoulders of the road were rough, just dirt and stones. I was stationary waiting on my bike on the dirt and off to the side of the road, with my back towards the on-coming traffic.

Unfortunately a lady accidentally drove her car off the bitumen and hit me at speed from behind. The force tossed both me and my bike up into the air, somersaulting onto her car bonnet and then rolling and crashing to road. In those days, cars had a long steel antenna which sliced open my left eyelid and down my face (I was just a hair's breadth away from losing my left eye).

Fortunately an off-duty policeman was in the following car and saw the whole thing – he also administered crucial first aid while waiting for the ambulance. I was knocked unconscious, had multiple injuries and was placed in intensive care for several days, remaining in hospital for several weeks and taking even more weeks at home recovering. This accident had a huge impact on me physically – who knew it would also have another massive impact on my health nine years later!

So George had been right about the past trauma to my body and he started to work on correcting my structure. The treatment was quite painful as muscles and tendons were forcibly released and realigned. Today you would probably categorise George's treatment as deep tissue massage or osteopathic though a later business card listed him as a chiropractor. Even though I was used to pain, I squirmed on the table as he worked and after an hour or so, he was finished.

Because we had travelled so far George said he wanted to see me two more times before I went home so I ended up having three intense treatments in that first week. I was so sore and came out in bruises all over my body but instinctively I knew it was doing me good.

At the end of my third visit, Mum asked me how I was feeling as I walked towards our car. All of a sudden I realised, I was walking easily, in a straight line! This may not sound much to others, but for me in the last couple of months, I could only walk painfully on a curve. Mum and I were amazed that one week of treatment had already started positive change.

So my recovery from MS evolved firstly with the discovery of the importance of body structural correction and postural realignment in promoting effective body functioning and repair. While my body had been so contracted and contorted physically, its own healing and correction mechanisms were hampered and severely restricted. By bringing my body back into structural alignment and balance, body systems were able to recommence doing what they needed to do to restore proper health and function.

Around the same time, I was doing my own research about how to heal myself, I was determined that I was going to overcome my prognosis.

Luckily my university degree was in journalism which had given me solid research skills. I could also speed read and had the ability to go through large amounts of information to find the 'treasure' or important points.

Early on in my research, I was lucky to come across two small but so valuable books *Lady Cilento on Vitamin and Mineral Deficiencies* and *The Cilento Way*. Actually for all my library research, these books had belonged to my parents and were at home in my father's office.

Lady Cilento was my earliest female inspiration. She was amongst the first female doctors in Australia and wrote many health and medical articles with her husband Sir Raphael 'Ray' Cilento from August 1929 for the then *Brisbane Courier* newspaper. So by the time I found Lady Cilento's books she had been writing about health and vitamin supplements for more than 50 years!

These two books gave me the nutritional information that undoubtedly helped turn my health around. People now tend to think that healthy eating and taking vitamins and minerals is some new age thinking but it is mind blowing to me that in fact Lady Cilento and her colleagues and inspirations, such as Dr Linus Pauling (won the Nobel Prize twice), Dr Irwin Stone (author of *The Healing Factor*), Dr Frederick R Klenner (world authority on the clinical use of vitamin C) and Dr Robert F Cathart (famous orthopaedic surgeon) were using vitamins very successfully in their research, surgeries and clinics for multiple health conditions so many years ago.

So around the same time my MS symptoms had started to decrease as my body was brought back into proper alignment and balance, I started taking mega-doses of vitamin C powder with bioflavonoids (including hesperidin and rutin) because it was indicated in Lady Cilento's books as being useful in fighting viral, bacterial and arthritic type conditions. The bioflavonoids were important to assist in the fast assimilation by the body.

Unlike many other animals and living things, humans (like monkeys, guinea pigs and fruit bats) do not manufacture their own vitamin C. It cannot be stored in the body and so it has to be consumed regularly in order to survive. Lady Cilento writes:

> *Vitamin C is non-toxic, has no side effects, does not build up in the body and any surplus to the body's needs quickly passes out in the urine ... This vitamin protects the body by aiding the adrenal glands to produce cortisone, maintains the strength of all the 'cementing' substance between cells, stimulates production of antibodies against germs and the number and effectiveness of the white blood cell.*

The exact cause of MS is unknown (most likely there are multiple causes) but it is a degenerative disease of the central nervous system. The MS Society (UK) advises that the immune system, which normally fights infections and protects the body, starts attacking and damaging the coating or myelin around the nerve fibres creating lesions or plagues which then disrupts crucial signals and smooth functioning between the brain and the rest of the body. Damage to the actual nerves can occur as well as myelin loss and this can create a variety of symptoms which tend to increase over time. To this day there is no definitive cure.

So from my research, I knew that MS was neurological and was caused by problems in the myelin sheath and nerve conduction but since my doctors could not help me, I decided that I need to try to rebuild my myelin and strengthen my body through vitamin supplementation in addition to the important corrective bodywork. Mega-doses of vitamin C were the corner stone of my personal attack on MS.

In his book *Food as Medicine*, Dr Earl Mindell advises:

> *Vitamin C, which is water-soluble, is essential for the formation of collagen, the substance that binds together the cells of connective tissue. Collagen is necessary for the production and growth of new cells and tissues: it also prevent viruses from penetrating the cell membrane ... it is especially important in the healing process.*

And of course in an ideal unpolluted, uncontaminated world with ready access to fresh raw food, not genetically modified, organically grown so not exposed to pesticides and other toxic chemicals, we should get all our vitamin needs from our food. But for most people today if you are not able to grow your own food (and a variety of it) then you might like to consider high quality, food-based natural supplements (less expensive synthetic supplements are cheap for a reason and can just expose you to more chemicals and toxins).

My decision back then to use vitamin C supplementation to help repair and support my body is also supported by other doctors now such as Dr Carole Hungerford, who in her book *Good Health in the 21st Century* writes about how vitamin C assists in the production of neuropeptides (neurotransmitters) and in the repair and synthesis of collagen amongst many other important body functions and uses.

During my research in 1985, I'd also found another interesting quote in *The Cilento Way* contending that "Sodium ascorbate, or vitamin C, is the only antibiotic that will get rid of a virus."

Because I had no way of knowing definitively what had caused my MS (and my doctors did not know either), I decided that this strategy might also help with the possibility of a viral contribution, so another reason to use vitamin C.

Lady Cilento had also mentioned in her books the importance of a fresh food diet and staying away from sugar, soft drink etc. While I didn't consume too much sugar, up to that point, I had been a big consumer of diet soft drinks. In those days consumers did not know of the potential dangers.

In high school it had become the 'in thing' to have a can of diet soft drink (or soda) for lunch, no food. Diet soft drinks were the new trendy beverages of choice in Australia at that time. So as teenage girls wanting to stay thin, we'd stand around in our lunch break (had no energy to do much else) slowly sipping our drink and chewing on the straws – we were so hungry!

My diet soft drink habit continued at university and was then supplemented with heavy coffee drinking, particularly at assignment and exam times. As well as overloading on saccharin, I had unknowingly become addicted to caffeine. Later when I finished university studies, I decided to wean myself off coffee even though it was then, and still now, totally socially acceptable to be a caffeine addict. However going cold turkey was quite an unexpected and unpleasant experience.

I had excruciating migraines for three days and all over body aches, etc. Needless to say having gone through caffeine withdrawal once, I have a very healthy respect for its powerful addictive effects. I now mostly drink organic herbal teas or an occasional water-decaffeinated organic coffee.

But during that same period there was little information in Australia about the dangers of consuming artificial sweeteners and diet soft drinks, and so I continued to drink them until my MS diagnosis. However I then followed Lady Cilento's writings and eliminated them completely from my diet.

Studies since then as noted in Sally Fallon's book, *Nourishing Traditions*, have indicated that the sugar, artificial sweeteners and phosphoric acid, etc., in soft drinks can have a negative impact on bones and joints. Elaine Hollingsworth in *Take Control of Your Health and Escape the Sickness Industry* contends that artificial sweeteners are a major cause of MS. I strongly feel my recovery was greatly assisted by eliminating the consumption of diet soft drinks.

I had learned a lot from my research and had taken immediate action to have as many physical treatments I could manage and to clean up my diet plus supplementing with high quality vitamin C powder (with bioflavonoids). My focus and determination was very high and of course I was buoyed by a decrease in my MS symptoms from that first week of corrective treatments.

My next visit was a month later when my mother and I drove down to see George, for three treatments again in the one week. This time at the end of the treatments, a second and most distressing symptom started to decrease – the fireworks and lightning. By the evening of that sixth treatment, the light show that had been constantly firing in my vision for many months, just disappeared! That night was the first time in a long time that I slept normally. Thankfully that light show never came back!

My pain levels were also decreasing and I was now able to walk normally up and down stairs (though initially very slowly and carefully). Once movement became easier, I wanted to continue to improve and keep moving. I began gentle exercise and yoga at home. I practiced meditation most days and made a conscious effort to keep thinking and speaking positively.

So it was with great excitement later back in Rockhampton, that I went to see my neurologist for the scheduled follow-up visit. I bounced into his office and told him how two of my major MS symptoms had disappeared with corrective bodywork and my use of superior nutrition and vitamin C. My neurologist was literally struck dumb.

I was obviously much better, not hobbling in on a walking stick or in a wheelchair as he had predicted. He took a couple of seconds before feebly insisting that I definitely did have MS and that there was no cure.

In an effort to help his other patients, I enthusiastically suggested that he might like to recommend they try bodywork and that it may also help them, but again he did not say much. I hope that he did think about that information and considered using it with his other patients, but I have no way of knowing as I never went back to see him again. I had no reason.

I continued to travel regularly to see George and stay for the week (having three treatments) for about a year. However within the first four months of doing that, eating fresh food, no white sugar, soft drink or artificial sweeteners, taking vitamin C plus gradually getting back into exercise, yoga and meditation, every MS symptom disappeared and I was able to return to full-time work.

Years have passed and my good health continues to this day. I still use those strategies to maintain my health but occasionally I stray. Life has a way of testing the best intentions. I've also found other tools to support my health (refer to Chapter Six and Ten) which help make up for the fact that I don't do everything perfectly all the time. Now I am a health warrior committed to the happiness and longevity of my family and clients.

For many years, I never spoke to friends or family about my battle with MS. By nature I'm a private person and don't like to dwell on the past or keep reviewing it. However when I began working as a therapist, I found in clinic the lessons I had learned from that particular period in my life were invaluable in assisting others with *any type of pain* (not just MS).

Personally experiencing that intense pain, fear and anger allowed me to develop a rapport and to really understand and help my clients. In fact the vast majority of my clientele come because of other health issues such as sporting injuries; accident recovery; back, leg and foot pain; neck and shoulder issues, headaches; migraines; posture imbalances; arthritic conditions; respiratory issues and stress etc. I've decided to share my story now in the hopes that it will help even more people outside my clinic situation.

Logically, in order to deal with any health condition, it is important to consider what caused it and then ideally rectify those issues. There are multiple causes and symptoms of MS so if that is your particular health battle, you may or may not be facing similar circumstances that I did. Looking back and knowing what I know now, I believe that *my* MS was triggered by three main issues:

1. Physical structural or postural abnormalities caused by my traumatic accident at the age of 13. Those structural imbalances were not diagnosed or treated at the time. Even to this day, many in the medical profession do not understand the importance or long-term impact of physical trauma and structural imbalance in the body.

   Of course when accidents occur, the more obvious and life-threatening symptoms such as fractures and bleeding, internal injuries, etc., have to take priority and thank goodness for the skills of our first responders and our wonderful doctors, emergency hospital and surgical staff. But when all the urgency and drama is over, the body's structural imbalance is rarely considered or corrected. In my case, this imbalance untreated at the time of my accident, had catastrophic effects years later. I also see similar situations regularly with my clients who have numerous health issues which resolve with structural correction.

2. The regular consumption of artificial sweeteners and high caffeine (in coffee and soft drinks, etc.) which was discussed earlier in this chapter (and in Chapter Six).

3. The emotional trauma of losing my father only ten months previously. That combined with severe structural imbalances meant that my body was struggling to cope both physically and emotionally. Back then there was also no recognition of the impact of emotional trauma, but now there are several ways of dealing with those stresses such as bodywork (eg., Bowen Therapy, reflexology and massage), Thought Field Therapy (TFT), yoga, meditation, positive visualisations, hypnosis, etc., which are discussed in later chapters of this book.

So Here's the Truth!

•   Sometimes severe or chronic pain is the wake-up call you need to kick yourself into immediate action. We can get complacent with our health and think we can just take a pill and fix everything. That is not always the case, sometimes *you* have to step up and take urgent action to fix the situation.

•   If you also get a bad diagnosis, you'll probably go through grief stages such as shock, denial, sadness and anger. You can use an emotive feeling such as anger to energise and fuel your fight back. Those strong feelings can focus and prod you into becoming your own health warrior and fighting – for yourself and your loved ones!

•   You always have a choice. Whatever your pain condition, you can choose to get a second (or a third) opinion. The medical profession is so specialised that people can be experts in their own field but have little knowledge of alternatives outside their expertise. Medical professionals are also often overworked and are looking after numerous patients who are all unique. Sometimes they don't have all the information needed to make the best decision (so do your part and always keep them fully informed) and occasionally test results are misinterpreted. There is a reason the term 'medical opinion' is widely used.

- Finally sometimes you, and everyone around you, can do everything right and you still get a bad outcome or no improvement in your pain. Sometimes bad things happen to good people but that's life and beyond our control. It is still important to never give up because you only fail when you stop trying!

CHAPTER 2

The Power of Pain!

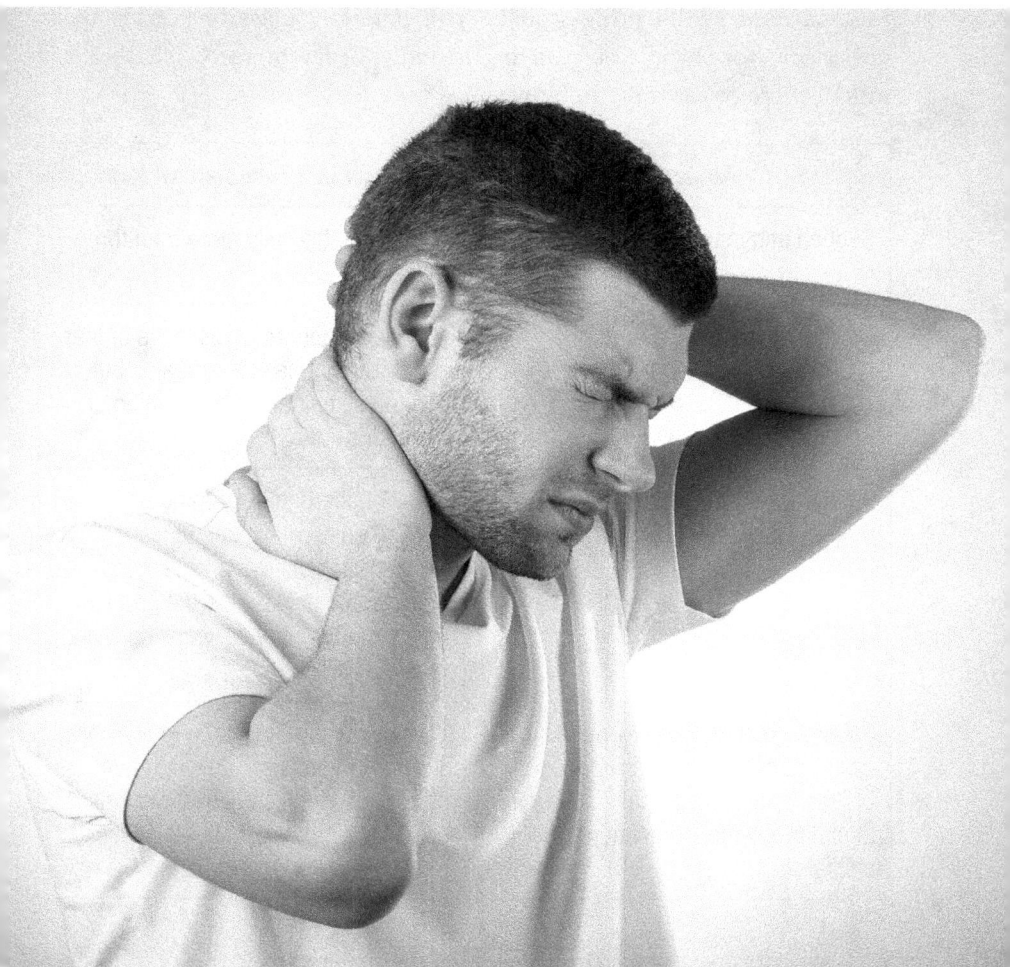

CHAPTER 2

The Power of Pain!

Pain is a warning sign that will tend to amplify in duration and intensity if the cause is not addressed. Of course you can mask the symptoms with medication and that may work successfully for some conditions or be effective for a long time. But ultimately for chronic pain getting to the cause and dealing with it, is really the solution for living pain free!

Medical and health professionals will generally classify your pain as either acute or chronic but *you* are the judge of its intensity, whether it is mild, severe or anything in between.

Acute Pain	Chronic (or persistent) Pain
Sudden and usually short term.	Long term, typically more than three months.
Normal response to trauma.	May be an abnormal response in that initial trauma may have healed but pain persists. Can be a condition or disorder by itself.
Sharp, aching or throbbing pain which may worsen on movement.	A mix of sharp, dull, burning or tingling pain, often experienced frequently or daily and includes neuropathic pain where the problem may be in the nerves, spinal cord or brain.
Cause is known, typically resulting from trauma to body tissue eg., broken bones, burns, cuts, surgery, dental problems, pregnancy and childbirth.	Cause may or may not be known. May result from ongoing, degenerative, musculoskeletal, infective, malignant conditions or no identifiable cause.

Acute Pain	Chronic (or persistent) Pain
Expected symptoms as per the trauma identified. Physiological signs such as wincing, grimacing, sweating, rapid pulse and breathing etc., which go away with healing.	Varied symptoms eg., headaches, back pain, joint or arthritic pain, nerve pain, tight muscles, limited mobility, tiredness, anxiety, anger, depression, fear, etc. Pain receptors may become hypersensitive and too easily activated or the brain and spinal cord may be unable to dampen or decrease pain signals.
Pain usually disappears when cause is treated or healed.	Pain persists after normal injury healing time or there may be no known cure.
If not treated effectively can develop into a chronic pain.	Referred pain and compensation patterns often develop.

Acute pain is typically caused by muscle, nerve or tissue damage as a result of trauma, injury or surgery. Since the reason is obvious, it is normally relatively easy to correct or remove the source of the pain. Accordingly acute pain will tend to decrease over time as the tissue damage heals or the source of pain is removed.

Unresolved pain that persists past three months is termed chronic and continues beyond the normal healing time. Its cause may not always be attributed to physical tissue damage. Chronic pain can also be the result of a degenerative or malignant condition or may have no readily identifiable origin.

Chronic pain activates the sympathetic nervous system, the body's 'fight or flight' automatic response. It places the body in continual stress mode which can impact on issues such as heart rate and blood pressure, constrict blood vessels, etc. It is not good for the body to remain in that heightened stress response. In *The Bowen Technique*, John Wilks writes:

The longer pain persists, the more scope there is for referred pain, for compensation patterns to be set up, and that it will spread and become more entrenched. When there is a level of inflammation in the tissues, which is nearly always the case, chronic pain will affect not only the peripheral nerves and the spinal cord, making them hypersensitive, but it will also have an activating effect on the sympathetic nervous system.

We can see from the following diagram that there are many factors which can contribute to the pain cycle.

CHRONIC PAIN CYCLE

Specialised nerve cells (nociceptors) send pain signals through the peripheral sensory nerves to the spinal cord and then the brain (thalamus) for processing and response in the somatosensory cortex (sensation), frontal cortex (thinking) and limbic system (emotional)

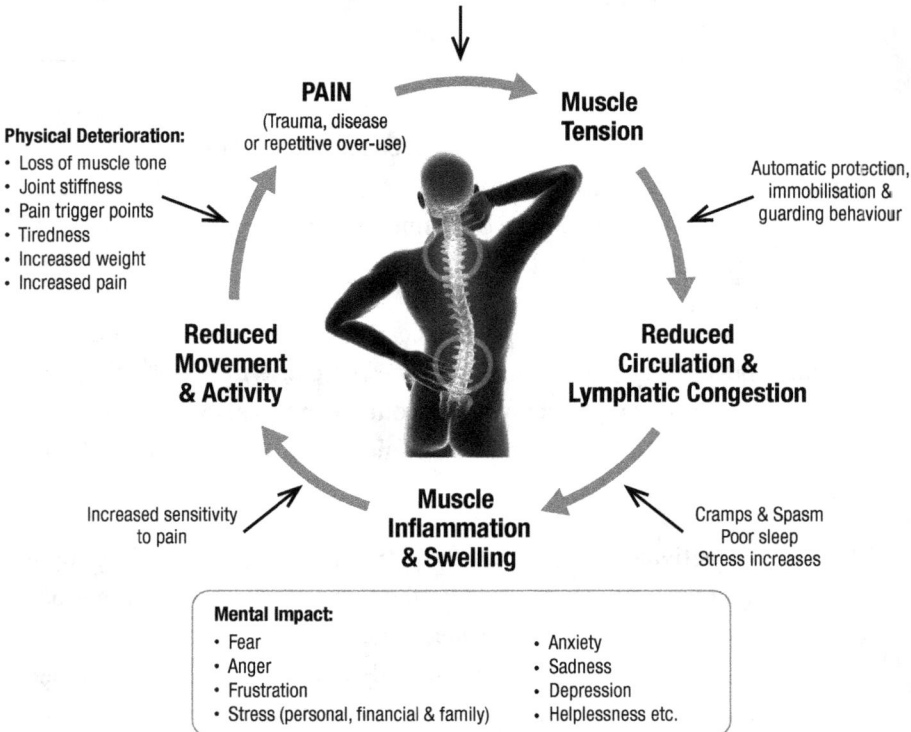

PAIN
(Trauma, disease or repetitive over-use)

Muscle Tension

Automatic protection, immobilisation & guarding behaviour

Physical Deterioration:
• Loss of muscle tone
• Joint stiffness
• Pain trigger points
• Tiredness
• Increased weight
• Increased pain

Reduced Movement & Activity

Reduced Circulation & Lymphatic Congestion

Increased sensitivity to pain

Muscle Inflammation & Swelling

Cramps & Spasm
Poor sleep
Stress increases

Mental Impact:
• Fear
• Anger
• Frustration
• Stress (personal, financial & family)
• Anxiety
• Sadness
• Depression
• Helplessness etc.

Did you know that pain is processed in the brain? I'm not being dismissive or saying that it is imaginary but from an anatomical and physiological point of view, pain is evaluated and processed in the brain (via the spinal cord). As chronic pain continues and progresses, negative changes can occur in the central nervous system and pain signals can be reinforced and continue to remain active even when not necessarily triggered and a hypersensitivity can develop. Painaustralia advises:

> *Chronic pain is associated with neuroplastic changes in the nervous system at peripheral, spinal cord and brain levels. Thus chronic pain is shown to have a distinct pathology that often worsens over time.*

The human brain is very clever at conserving energy and conscious attention by continually learning, strengthening and reinforcing nerve pathways and learned behaviours, so repetitive actions, thoughts and emotions can easily become habitual and require no conscious effort. While great for learning a sport or new skill, this ability can be massively detrimental in long-term pain conditions.

Anything that you practice or repeat frequently whether it is a thought, emotion, action or reaction can become an ingrained and habitual response. This can also happen with pain signals to the brain. With chronic pain, because of repeated stimulation and reinforcement, nerve pathways transmitting pain messages to the brain can become entrenched and easily triggered.

Neuroplasticity or brain plasticity is a fast developing field of research that has implications for pain management. Contrary to previous medical belief, the brain has now been found to be able to form new neural connections and reorganise itself even into adulthood. So the brain can form and grow new nerve connections to compensate for disease or trauma.

In the book *The Brain That Changes Itself*, Dr Norman Doidge lists numerous studies which prove the wonderful pliability and plasticity of the human brain and how repeated thoughts and actions can actually rewire nerve pathways. This is why people with brain injury can restore body function by using different parts of the brain and establishing and developing new neural pathways.

It then follows that it is possible to train or use the brain to process pain signals differently and therefore relieve pain. We just have to learn how to stop using those ingrained neural pathways. And while I am not saying it is easy, it certainly is possible.

Supporting this concept of training the brain to relieve pain, a recent American trial of 342 adults with chronic lower back pain, results of which were published in the *Journal of the American Medical Association*, found that those who did meditation and yoga obtained more effective pain relief than those that undertook more traditional treatment. Dr Daniel Cherkin, from the Group Health Research Institute in Seattle, Washington, reported that:

> *Pain and other forms of suffering involve the mind as well as the body ... research suggests that training the brain to respond differently to pain signals may be more effective – and last longer – than traditional physical therapy and medication.*

Obviously pain is complex and multifaceted. Social or psychological factors can also impact on chronic pain conditions. Dr Bruce Lipton in *The Biology of Belief* reports that people in a loving, supportive and social environment will tend to deal with pain more positively and heal more quickly than those who are alone or in a non-supportive environment.

Research also found that certain genes can be changed and look markedly different in people who are alone versus those who have a large social network. The affected gene pool also has important roles in inflammatory immune responses which then has an impact on pain and may also effect associative diseases such as atherosclerosis and depression.

Resultant depression from chronic pain should not be taken lightly. According to Painaustralia:

> *One in five Australian adults with severe or very severe pain also suffer depression or other mood disorders ... if left untreated can lead to suicide. Like depression, chronic pain can become a serious and debilitating disease in its own right. It can significantly diminish quality of life for patients and their families and the risk of suicide is twice as high in people who have chronic pain.*

So please seek professional help if you are struggling with that situation. Some useful contacts are also listed in the Recommended Resources section at the back of this book.

Just as there are multiple factors that can contribute to your pain condition, there are numerous ways that it is typically treated. Your doctor may prescribe painkillers such as non-steroidal anti-inflammatory drugs (NSAIDs) or opioid pain relievers/narcotics such as morphine or codeine. You might be offered surgery, nerve blocks, physical therapy, psychotherapy and/or rehabilitation etc. Usually those strategies work well, however there are times they do not. In the next chapters, I detail some complementary natural therapies and techniques that work well with those traditional strategies and can give you some more fire power to win the battle over pain!

Here's the Truth!

- You already know personally what pain is and how it can make you feel. It can keep grinding you down until you find it hard to remember a time when you weren't in great pain. You despair of ever feeling good again and anxiety or depression can start to raise its ugly head.

- You also probably know how at first people sympathised with you but as the days dragged on into weeks and months, they began to get tired of you and your pain because while it exhausts you, it also exhausts those around you. Then people start to avoid you and slowly you become isolated and lonely in your pain.

- But you can fight back and you don't have to continue to accept your current situation. You can get angry about it and totally annoyed with the unfairness of it all but then decide to use that anger. After all anger is just an emotion or 'energy in motion'. So you can choose to use that energy in positive ways to your advantage, to motivate and become determined to conquer your pain. You have to dig deep but your power is there, just patiently waiting for you to step up and use it!

On a personal note, when I was diagnosed, pain medications did not work for me and a big motivation at that time was finding relief. If my pain meds had worked, I may have sat back passively, accepted my diagnosis and would probably have rapidly deteriorated and passed away just as my neurologist predicted. Now when I look back, my pain was actually my saviour!

And so this is the power of pain. Once you become determined to fight and overcome it, you have a mission and a different focus, a distraction from your pain and then it becomes your powerful motivation. Because frankly the vast majority of us will do anything to avoid pain.

Then once you overcome it, you will become so empowered and strong. You will come to know that it is not a permanent condition and that you can beat it – you just have to engage the fighter, awaken the warrior in you.

> *"Pain does not have to mean suffering, it can actually be the birth of a stronger and more powerful you."*
>
> **Suzanne McTier-Browne**

CHAPTER 3

The Power of Correcting Body Alignment

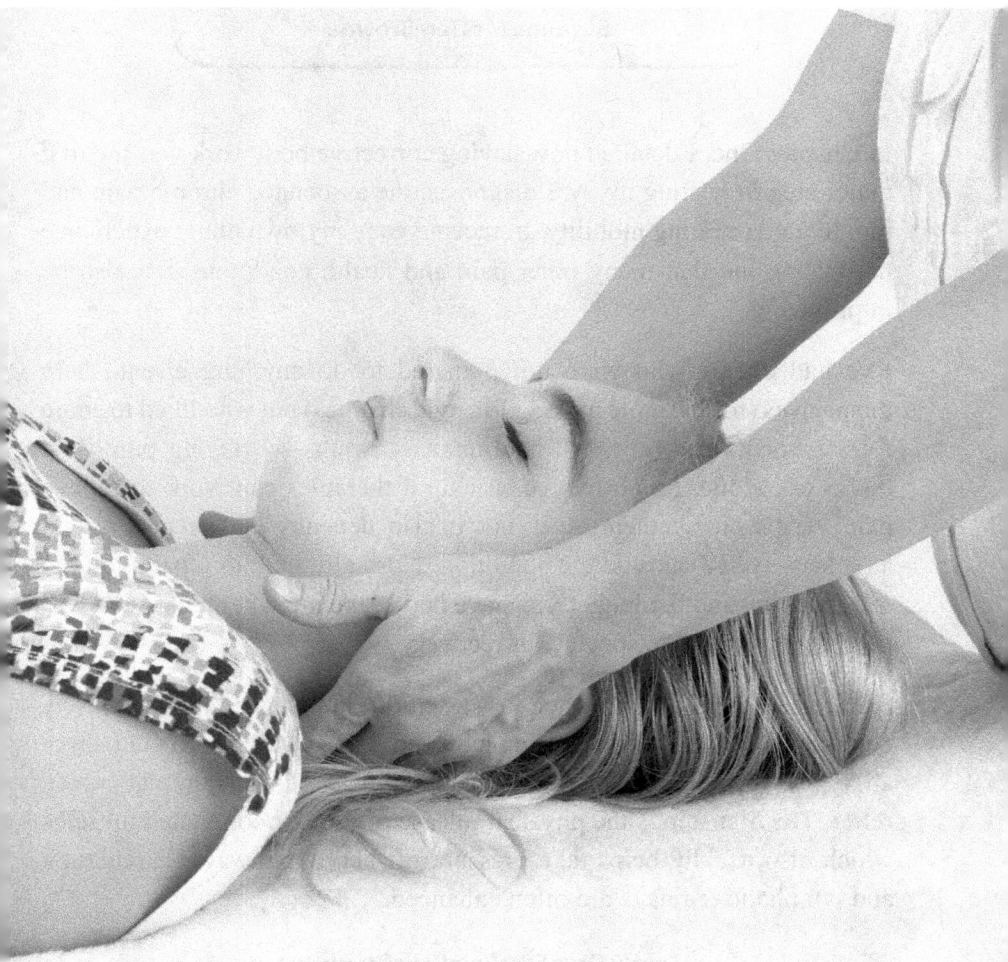

CHAPTER 3

The Power of Correcting Body Alignment

> *"Correcting posture and restoring proper body alignment can be the most important factor in becoming pain free and staying that way."*
>
> **Suzanne McTier-Browne**

In Chapter One, I detailed how having corrective bodywork was the first major step in beating my MS diagnosis, the associated chronic pain and rapidly deteriorating mobility. In recent years, my own clinic experience has shown me that many other pain and health conditions can also be improved.

I've had clients who were not prepared to do anything else to help themselves (for example making lifestyle changes) but who liked to come for treatments and they still had amazing results by relying purely on bodywork alone. So corrective structural therapies can work to relieve pain very well by themselves but it also depends on the person and how serious and chronic the condition. Normally the more pain you are experiencing and the longer you have had it, the more strategies you will need to implement to speed your recovery.

Also, please note that when a structural imbalance and/or muscle contraction in the body is causing pain and it needs to be corrected, there are typically three steps or phases that are processed through to gain pain relief. The first step is the physical release of tight or contracted muscles which also usually helps take pressure off nerve pathways. Circulation and lymphatic drainage are often enhanced.

Because muscles attach to bones, in the second step, that physical release then allows the bony structure or skeleton to rebalance and make minor adjustments and corrections. The final third phase is that with the body structure more balanced, function and mobility are also improved and there begins a reduction in the triggering and firing of nerves, and so pain decreases. Depending on the person and their pain condition, this three-phase pain relief after physical structural correction may happen very quickly or can take several days to process.

Bowen Therapy

An Australian physical therapy, the Bowen Technique, was developed by the late Tom Bowen (1916–1982). I had already qualified as a massage therapist prior to studying Bowen Therapy and found it to be such an intelligent, unique and beautifully gentle way of correcting structure and posture while working with the body to achieve healthy balance and function.

Since I already had a working knowledge of anatomy and physiology and had developed a 'tissue sense', I could see and feel the changes in the client as we did the Bowen moves. Tissue sense is an ability that a therapist can develop from experience and working on people – just by placing hands on a person or through gentle palpation, extra information can be gained about circulation, contraction in muscle fibres, hydration, etc. Not all therapists develop that skill so when you are looking for someone to be on your team to help you with your pain, perhaps try and find someone with that extra ability.

It was amazing to see and feel the muscles release on the table after the Bowen moves, and that was just the first day! Because I was so aware of its potential in helping relieve the suffering of others, I accelerated my training. Finally I'd found a therapy that could give similar results to what I had experienced all those years ago. A bonus was that it was so gentle while still being profoundly effective.

Around this time, I received a phone call from a local doctor. A couple of her patients had seen me for pain relief and told of their positive results.

Dr Jo Turner offered me a room at The Family Medical Practice. Not many people then knew about Bowen and here was a far-sighted doctor, with the benefit of her patients in mind, inviting me to join her clinic. The years I worked there with Dr Turner and the other doctors greatly increased my exposure to clients with various pain conditions. Still to this day it amazes me with the improvements that can be achieved with Bowen Therapy even if clients have tried everything else.

Basically, Bowen has given me the tools to assist thousands of clients, and to be able to help someone gently without adding trauma is wonderful. While more forceful body therapies are also valuable, with the gentleness of Bowen, I've found that the body does not go into defence or protection mode, so muscles do not tighten up and the body is not further stressed.

People who are in pain or have been traumatised, are already in sympathetic stress or in 'fight or flight' which can increase pain and hamper recovery. Bowen has the unique ability to switch off that stress switch and place the body into parasympathetic mode, instantly calming the body and letting the focus be on pain relief and healing.

Bowen is an intelligent way of de-stressing the body, taking the pressure and contraction out of muscles and joints so that the body can relax and repair. And while many people come to Bowen for assistance with musculoskeletal issues, from my personal and clinic experience, it has potential to help with so many other conditions including being useful before surgery. It enables the body to be in the best physical and structural condition before going into surgery and then helps with healing and recovery afterwards.

I have required numerous surgeries throughout the years and always found that a visit with Suzanne for a Bowen treatment pre- and post-surgery to release pressure and tight muscles and to improve circulation would always assist in pain relief and improve my recovery time. Thank you Suzanne.   Taneya S.

The added beauty of Bowen is that it is complementary and can work well with existing conventional medical treatment. It is a gentle and safe therapy that can help with muscular, structural problems and the pain associated with:

✓ Sport injuries   ✓ Migraines & headaches

✓ Accident recovery   ✓ Circulation problems

✓ Back pain & sciatica   ✓ Abnormal posture

✓ Leg, knee & foot problems ✓ Constipation

✓ Sinus & Asthma   ✓ Hormonal problems

✓ Stress & tension   ✓ Body detoxification

✓ Neck & shoulder problems and so much more!

Bowen is also wonderful for strengthening, maintenance and prevention programs. I personally have regular Bowen sessions to keep me going through the busy times and operating at the top of my game. I also have many hard-working business professionals as clients who have regular Bowen to relieve their pain, reduce stress and the possibility of downtime from injury or illness. There are also huge benefits for athletes. In *Bowen Unravelled*, Julian Baker writes:

> *Bowen is a particularly effective treatment for long-term sports injury prevention. Athletes being treated with Bowen report remarkable responses in terms of fewer injuries, as well as faster recovery after minor injuries.*

My athlete clients come from a variety of sports such as athletics, swimming, basketball, football, tennis, martial arts, gymnastics, trampolining, gym, dancing, yoga and crossfit. Because they have great muscle tone, they usually respond quickly.

I am a crossfit fanatic which involves weight work and cardio, jumping and running. I go to crossfit four or five times a week. I participate in in-house competitions and I hate being hampered by injury or pain.

In August 2015 I injured my right ankle/foot and was unable to do any running, weighted squats or box jumps. I started weekly treatment in massage and dry needling. By December of the same year my left hip started causing me problems (due to compensating for the injury in my foot). This turned out to be bursitis, causing me extreme pain and now I was unable to climb stairs without heavily supporting myself. I gave up on massage and dry needling as I was getting no relief at all.

In February 2016 I started regular weekly treatment with a physio. Nine months later – still in a lot of pain and with no relief whatsoever I gave up. I was still unable to run and participate in a lot of exercises at crossfit and to make matters worse, walking was also becoming difficult.

After having absolutely no relief, I contacted Suzanne in November 2016. I was quite a mess with extreme pain in my right foot/ankle and hip. Lying on my left side was now almost impossible as the pressure on my hip was very painful. I had three sessions quite close to try and sort out this pain.

What can I say – within these three treatments (yes three) I was starting to move more freely. I still struggled a bit and was still unable to run. However, walking had become a lot easier and I was starting to climb the steps a bit more freely, with only minimal support.

I had another Bowen Therapy session towards the end of April. About two weeks later I decided to participate in a fitness test at the gym and for the first time since injuring my ankle/foot and hip I was able to complete a 1 km run. I was over the moon. I certainly wished I had received Bowen Therapy right from the start. I am now also able to box jump and complete weighted squats.

> So, all up I've had four sessions of Bowen Therapy. I have had more pain relief and movement returned to me in 4 sessions than all the months of massage, dry needling and physio ever did.
>
> I highly recommend Bowen and Suzanne for relief of chronic pain and immobility.   Debbie A.

Part of my goal with this book is to educate people about some powerful natural therapies and techniques they can use in their pain relief journey. Bowen Therapy has been available for many years now but it's still relatively new to many people. Now the word is getting out! *Healthy Soul* in the UK reports that a number of celebrities and sportspeople have used Bowen including Kylie Minogue, Elle Macpherson and James Ellison. It quotes Bear Grylls:

> *Bowen has helped keep my body together despite the continual bashing it takes. It's a vital support in putting right a whole range of new aches and pains, making sure that old injuries don't cause me problems, and helping me fight stress and fatigue.*

James Ellison, British Superbike Champion, also talks about his experience with Bowen Therapy:

> *I have never felt so good and will continue to recommend it to anyone looking for pain relief or even just wanting to improve their quality of life.*

As well as adults, the elderly and athletes, children and babies benefit enormously from Bowen Therapy. Babies can safely be worked on from birth.

> Shelby started being unsettled about three weeks and waking in between feeds to vomit or burp and cry in pain. At six weeks, she often refused to feed. Shelby now seems much more comfortable and sleeps for longer periods without becoming restless or even waking. Doesn't refuse to feed. She has had three weekly treatments to date. They do not hurt her and I find her much more relaxed for days after. I thoroughly recommend Bowen Therapy and Suzanne you are a lovely person who put my mind at rest when I was looking into getting help for my beautiful baby girl. Thank you.
>
> Brenda C. & Shelby (ten weeks).

My clinic experience, having helped over 2,000 clients and completing more than 10,000 sessions, has proven to me how valuable Bowen Therapy can be. Hopefully the testimonials and case studies in this book will encourage you to try your local therapist.

But as much as I love Bowen Therapy and it works wonderfully for so many people, the universe kept sending me extremely complex cases and so I was continually on the search for extra information and techniques that could help my clients.

Reflexology

I became a Reflexologist in 2004, a really useful therapy that has a long history (around 5,000 years) in Chinese, Egyptian and Indian medicine. In 1582, two European doctors published a book on zone therapy and British neurologist, Sir Henry Head in the 1890s, identified skin or head zones that corresponded to internal organs.

Modern reflexology then developed in the west, largely based upon the work of American Dr William Fitzgerald, known as the founder of zone therapy, and Eunice Ingham, the Mother of Modern Reflexology. In the late 1800s and early 1900s, many doctors used reflexology or zone techniques for pain relief. However, like most bodywork, it can be time consuming so as doctors needed to help larger numbers of people and drugs became popular, those body skills were mostly let go.

Reflexology primarily addresses the foundation of the body, the feet (although it also has wonderful applications with the hands, ears and face). Like a house or building, if the foundations are not sound or are structurally unbalanced it can have a detrimental influence on the integrity of the rest of the structure. Like Bowen Therapy, it also deals with the body's fascia, circulation, lymphatic and central nervous systems.

Because areas of the body have associated reflexes in the feet (and the hands, ears and face), it enables a therapist to help someone who is uncomfortable with physical touch to the body or allows support for an injured area that cannot be worked on directly.

Nature & Health magazine reports that in a double-blind trial, migraine patients given reflexology found it as effective as Flunarizine drug therapy. And children suffering from chronic constipation given reflexology had significant reductions in their pain scores.

Babies can also benefit from reflexology. Baby Reflex, currently available in England, Australia, South Africa, Abu Dhabi, Eire, Northern Ireland, Scotland, Wales, Japan, Turkey and Europe, is a gentle form of reflexology created especially for babies (from one month), infants and toddlers. It aims to calm, ease discomfort and improve sleep patterns. Developed by Jenny Lee, a Physiotherapist and Reflexologist, Baby Reflex gives parents the opportunity to learn special, gentle, techniques which they can use at home. Empowering for parents who can adjust the treatment to suit their own child's needs.

If pain means that it is difficult for you to be touched or get up and then down off a massage table, reflexology can provide further treatment options as it can be done in a chair or on a bed. Hands, ears or face can be worked if feet are not an option. (Bowen can also be done seated or in a wheelchair.)

There are really no excuses for you not to try quality bodywork in support of relieving your pain. Finding long term relief is your most important investment. Once you are pain free consider a maintenance program to keep you enjoying life at your physical best.

> *"Your body is your most precious asset – invest in high quality bodywork regularly. You deserve a life without pain!"*
>
> **Suzanne McTier-Browne**

Massage

Remedial and deep-tissue massage uses strong pressure on tight and contracted areas and concentrates on releasing deeper layers of muscle. Techniques can include cross fibre, trigger point release, stretching and it's useful for muscle pain, sporting and occupational injuries, injury rehabilitation, body tension and stress.

The American Massage Therapy Association reports that several studies have shown that massage therapy may be effective for chronic low-back pain and may decrease reliance on anti-inflammatory drugs, particularly when combined with exercise and rehabilitation. Massage may also assist with conditions such as arthritis, neck pain and fibromyalgia.

Massage, Bowen and reflexology are professional government accredited courses in Australia and also require extensive studies in anatomy and physiology. However, just like there are good and bad practitioners in any profession, there can be big quality and experience differences between therapists. You quickly learn who knows what they are doing and those who don't, are bluffing and really should just get a different job.

I've continued to have bodywork regularly myself and while I love having Bowen, reflexology and massage, I've also benefited from chiropractic treatment. I like to try different therapies and have had some excellent treatment along the way but have also experienced some not so great.

I've had people walking on my back and have been pinched, punched, pummelled and stretched into unusual positions that didn't help.

Sometimes the treatment actually caused injury. Having had some negative experiences in the past, I now only go to government accredited practitioners and price is not a factor – you get what you pay for!

Usually when I am travelling, I try to get a massage or local treatment for research and to keep functioning at my best while away on business. One time, I decided to try a massage franchise near my hotel in Brisbane. The lady on the desk spoke excellent English and the sign said the therapists were accredited so I thought it would be ok – boy was I wrong!

I was led into a small, cramped and not very clean massage cubicle. I lay face down on the table and the young lady started flopping her hand on my back. I could tell it was just one hand and this unusual move was also highly ineffective. I waited for half a minute but the 'dying fish' flopping technique continued, so slightly irritated I lifted my head off the table to see the therapist (and I use the term lightly as obviously she was not trained at all) was texting on her mobile phone with the other hand. She was startled and jumped when I looked at her. I told her that I was finished and got off the table, I didn't want someone untrained, unskilled and uninterested working on me.

Her English was extremely poor and obviously not an Australian trained therapist at all, even though the receptionist had told me that she would be. So now I'm very careful when having treatments that I get someone who has completed government accredited training in Australia or some other country with comparable standards.

So the first and most important thing to do is to find yourself a great musculoskeletal therapist with whom you feel confident and comfortable. Make sure they are a member of a professional association which ensures educational, training and ethical standards have been met. Listed in the Recommended Resources at the end of this book are the professional associations for the therapies mentioned. Also ask around, word of mouth can be a great resource. Continue to search until you've found the right person for you.

Do not be discouraged if you get little improvement after a few sessions with your first choice, just try someone else. Giving up on the first try says more about you than it does them. It's only failure if you stop trying – keep going until you succeed in finding the right therapist for you.

With chronic pain, a multipronged attack may work better and depending on your pain condition, you might benefit from using a couple of different therapists at different stages in your recovery. Typically the longer you have been dealing with your pain and the more complex your condition, the more effort it takes to recover and the more people you may need on your team. This is the time for you to be honest and to ask for help when you need it.

Of course, first port of call is generally your doctor who can take care of your tests, medications and referrals etc. Second, from my personal experience and results in clinic, you should consider finding yourself a good physical therapist to help correct any postural and structural misalignments and imbalances. You might consider adding a Bowen Therapist, Reflexologist, Massage Therapist or Chiropractor to your team.

Some people need more than one and have also benefited at times from alternating Bowen with chiropractic or massage for example. It's often wise to do only one therapy at a time so you can gauge what is working for you and you might find that one perfect therapist who is all you need. Perhaps start with a series of Bowen sessions and if that begins to plateau or stall in improvements, have a few visits with another health professional.

Another member in your team could be a Physiotherapist, Exercise Physiologist, Personal Trainer or Yoga Instructor to personalise your exercise and stretch plan. You might also consult a Naturopath or Homeopath. Often the different therapies deal with different issues, sometimes there is overlap. You might be lucky enough to find just one therapist who works brilliantly in several areas. Of course there are many other health professionals you could consider adding to your team.

Finally, if you are hesitating to try and invest in the therapies above, perhaps start thinking of your body as a prestige car. To ensure it runs efficiently and to enhance its performance, you would naturally book it in for regular services and maintenance. With care and attention, you can lengthen its lifespan.

Of course your body is so much more valuable! You may have several cars in your lifetime but only one body! We should care for ourselves at least as much and have regular services to keep our body running in peak condition. This strategy can also prevent high maintenance in the future. It is so much harder to regain good health once you've lost it!

With more than 2,000 clients, the variety of pain challenges they face is huge, and the vast majority have been impacted in very positive ways with Bowen Therapy, reflexology and massage. At the very least, no one has been hurt in the process and their circulation and lymphatic drainage has improved.

In health there is a basic principle that stagnation can lead to death (of tissue or the body), so anything that improves the body's circulatory system is generally a great thing. Poor circulation can also be a huge issue for pain and conditions such as diabetes, arthritis, sports injuries, etc. What do you have to lose? In my case, great bodywork improving circulation and function, as well as correcting structural alignment helped saved my life!

> *"Life is energy, movement and change, stagnation leads to deterioration, decline and death."*
>
> **Suzanne McTier-Browne**

CHAPTER 4

The Perils of Poor Posture

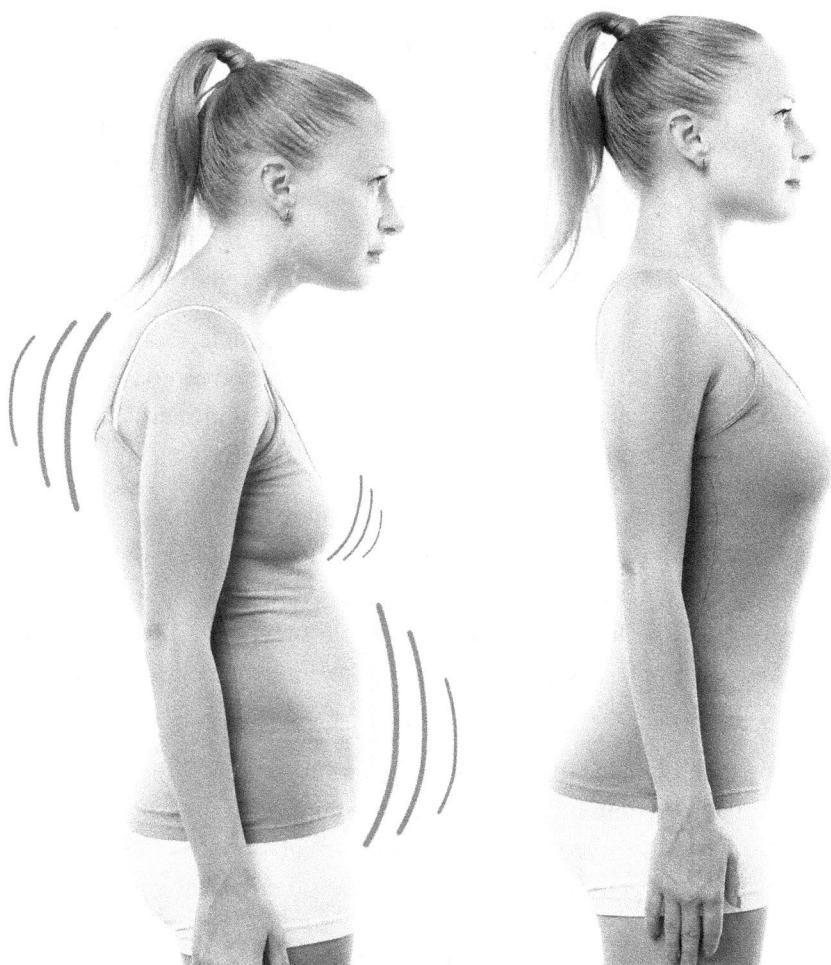

CHAPTER 4

The Perils of Poor Posture

Many of us over the age of 40 may remember being forced to stand to attention during school assembly on the parade ground while the national anthem was played. At my schools (both primary and high school) we had to stand for the whole assembly. We were made to stand up straight (no slouching allowed) and I remember being tapped on the back or head if I was stooped to remind me to stand at attention. In primary school, we had to sit up straight and weren't allowed to rest our elbows on the desk.

That seems to have all changed now, and not for the better. When my children went to school, I noticed at assembly that they either sat on the floor or in chairs. No teacher checked their posture and so all I saw was a mess of mostly slumped little bodies with rarely anyone sitting up straight. Of course, mobile phone and computer use now compounds the problem.

Over the last decade in clinic, I've seen a progressive deterioration in the overall posture and fitness of most children, unless they are into sport. The incidence of upper back and neck pain is increasing and many children have surprisingly limited range of motion in their necks.

They also often come with issues such as rounded shoulders, slumped posture and respiratory problems – do you think there might be a possible connection? Do you think the lungs can fully inflate and children can breathe easily if the head is down (constricting the throat and airway) and they are constantly slumped forward, crowding and compressing the lungs and organs in the trunk of the body?

It's sad to see children with poor muscle tone from very little exercise, constantly playing computer games and not going outside to run and play. They come with sore knees, hips, ankles and many are now flat footed. And while flat feet can be genetic, it can also be environmental. These issues can often be resolved with quality body structural correction, but it is a concern that young bodies are so stiff and in pain. In the past, this only used to happen to the elderly or those who had been in accidents.

Some children rarely go outside these days in bare feet, but as a Reflexologist, I can tell you that our feet were designed to bend and flex naturally as we walk, jump, balance and climb over various natural surfaces. Little time outside doing a variety of physical activities means that key muscles are not being strengthened or stretched.

Exercising outside and exposure to fresh air, sunlight (getting natural vitamin D), all help to strengthen bones and joints, of everyone not just children. And especially if you're battling pain or don't want it back again.

So now let's take a look at the following photos – which one is more like you?

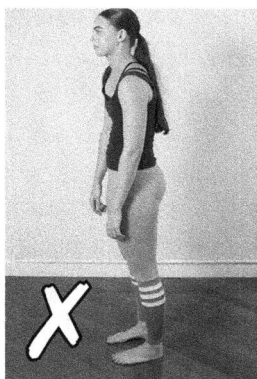

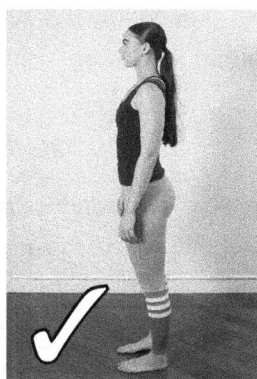

Can you see how in the 'bad' posture photo on the left, the rounded shoulders and upper back compress the chest, lungs, heart and the stomach tends to protrude because the organs in the trunk of the body are cramped and pushed together? This posture also forces the head and neck into abnormal posture and increases the pressure in those areas plus the throat and jaw.

The weight of the human head, around 5 kg or 11 pounds for an adult, is borne by the neck and shoulder muscles and if not aligned with the spine can create tightness and soreness. The more forward the head comes, the effective weight of it increases and more strain is created on the neck and shoulders.

Because breathing then becomes cramped and shallow, the body can go into stress mode and over time this creates tiredness and exhaustion (physical and mental). This continual posture can also create headaches, migraines, jaw clenching and temporomandibular joint (TMJ) syndrome, neck and shoulder pain (including between the shoulder blades), arm tingling and numbness, spinal deterioration and breathing discomfort.

> Having pneumonia affected all of my daily activities. I wasn't able to work or look after my family. It made me weak and unfit and my posture was quite bad. After my first Bowen treatment with Suzanne I felt I could breathe easier, I stood straighter and I was able to complete some more chores because I felt more energized. That particular night I even commented to my husband that I was feeling better.
> Brenda C.

However this 'lazy' posture does not only affect the upper body. Because everything is connected it can impact on the lower back and hips with the stomach protruding forward and the buttocks flattening. Circulation, lymphatic flow, digestion and the bowel can be affected and it can contribute to lower back ache and pelvic issues. If this posture is you, can you see how it might be contributing to your pain condition?

This is also an age accelerating posture. People with youth, physically or in their mental outlook, stand tall and straight and move freely and easily. A round shouldered, slumped posture is aging and contributes to premature deterioration of many body systems.

In the 'good' posture photo, you can see how the spine, neck and head is comfortably and vertically aligned. Once everything is aligned, there is little effort to maintain the correct posture so tiredness and lack of energy becomes less of an issue.

There is no compression or cramping in the chest so the lungs can expand freely for deep and relaxed breathing. There is no unnecessary pressure on the heart, stomach, throat, jaw or neck so they can work effectively without added stress. Overall movement is easier because of correct posture.

Now if you have had 'bad' posture for a while because of your pain or health condition, it will probably be difficult to improve your posture without assistance and this is where corrective bodywork, as discussed in Chapter Three, is invaluable. Once you have had tight muscles and pressure released from your body, you will find it easier to stand (and sit) with more correct posture. It is then up to you to practice and maintain good posture daily.

> *"Your body is like your house. If the foundations are misaligned or unsound, the structure above becomes weak and has to compensate to remain upright. This can set up pain patterns in the rest of the body."*
>
> **Suzanne McTier-Browne**

Preventative Pain Measures

If you are in pain, or even once you become pain free, you should be on the lookout for triggers in your environment. Some things to look out for:

- Have you heard the saying "sitting is the new smoking" – it's true! Sitting for too long or in the wrong position can have major pain consequences.

- If you work on computers frequently make sure the work space and layout *suits you*. Make sure that the monitor is at comfortable eye level so you don't have to tilt your head down and that the mouse is within easy reach (without over extending your arm/shoulder). Keep your head and spine vertically aligned – constantly tilting the head forward and down, tightens neck and shoulders muscles. Take frequent breaks to move freely and drink water!

- Your feet should be able to comfortably rest on the floor (or stool) and not swing from the seat. Maybe a 'Sit to Stand' or ergonomic desk may be the answer for you. Test personally before you buy if possible and select a good quality chair – if you have back and pain issues this is not the time to buy cheap.

- Poor phone posture – have you ever looked at someone (or yourself in the mirror) while using your mobile phone or tablet? Head forward and down, rounded upper back and shoulders – it's not a pretty sight. Prolonged texting, watching movies or using Facebook etc. helps create what was called years ago 'dowagers hump'.

Trauma or fractures can cause the condition but some people also get it from constant work with the head down; some from hormone issues and now many people, even teenagers, have it from poor posture. Unless you have spinal degeneration, fractures or fusing, it doesn't have to be that way. It doesn't have to continue and if caught early and with a bit of effort can be turned around. But a big first step is correcting that bad posture.

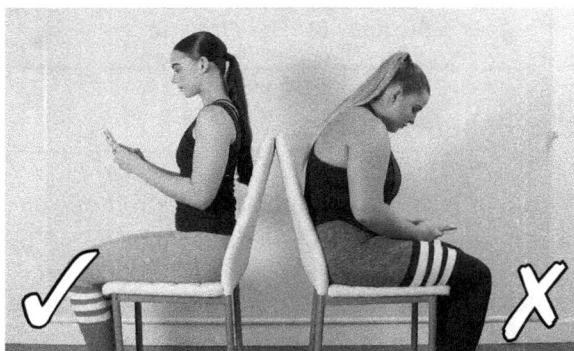

Some suggestions:

- For short periods of mobile phone or tablet usage, hold the device up to eye level, keeping your spine and neck straight as possible.

- For longer periods, you may need to prop your device on a stand or use it at the table or desk to get it close to your eye level and not have to tilt your head down. Be creative, do whatever it takes to use your device in a comfortable and good posture position.

> *"Pain is your wake-up call – don't keep doing activities that cause you distress. Protect yourself – be aware, assess your activities and then take action to amend."*
>
> **Suzanne McTier-Browne**

Become aware of bad furniture design. Often lounge and TV chairs are made to look good but they may not be the best for your back. They may tilt your back too far backwards and if they are too soft, you can really sink into the seating and then find it difficult to get up from that position. So while soft seems so inviting, in reality it may not be good for your bad back. I have multiple clients who have hurt themselves getting out of the lounge chair after falling asleep or jumping up in a rush to answer a phone or doorbell.

The ideal chair is one that allows you to keep your back relatively straight and vertically aligned – unlike this typical chair shown in the following photo. Generally you should be sitting slightly forward on your hips and tailbone not leaning backwards with your spine past vertical. Push your buttocks into the back of the chair so you are sitting upright.

Extend and pull up through your spine – don't sag into the chair and allow your rib cage to collapse onto your stomach and hips. Pull up through the crown of the head and rest your hands on mid thighs (not clasped together or crossed in front of your chest). Shoulders should be down and relaxed to help keep an open chest with your elbows hanging vertically.

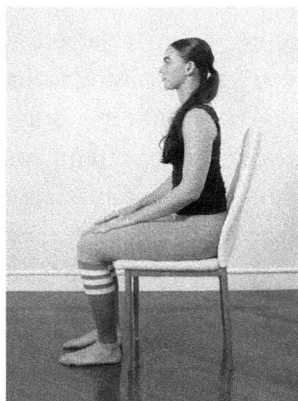

Chairs that tilt your spine back will make you (unconsciously) push your head and neck forward so that your body can find a centre point of gravity. Your body has an inbuilt balance mechanism that means when your body is tilted backwards, your head will automatically come forward to compensate. As soon as that happens, neck and shoulder muscles strain and tighten, circulation is affected and pain can be initiated or increased.

Most lounge chairs today are plush and you tend to sink deeply into the seat – I avoid those chairs because I know they can trigger my back and I want to stay pain free. Soft chairs can be a trap for people who end up sitting all day and maybe falling asleep in the chair. For many pain conditions, being 'lazy' and sitting all day can have painful consequences. If you have back issues, you should choose wisely how, where and how long you sit.

People also come with different leg and spine lengths so one chair design is not ideal for all. For example a too high chair can press on the hamstrings, the back of the legs of a shorter person and over time can compromise circulation and lymphatic drainage. This can result in tight calves and swelling of the feet and ankles. Pick a chair where your legs are not swinging but your feet comfortably reach the floor (or use a foot stool). Also flex your feet and stretch your legs regularly while seated to avoid circulation problems.

If you have back, hip or knee pain, and the length of the chair seat is too long, you may have difficulty getting out of the chair suddenly. Or if you've been sitting far back into a chair, do not stand up immediately from that position. First, bring yourself forward horizontally towards the front edge of the seat until you can get your feet firmly on the ground. Tighten your core or stomach muscles, lean slightly forward over your knees and then rise. Stand for a few seconds for your circulation to equalise and to regain your balance before you move away. Stop and visualise what you want to do next and then move – no need to rush. Do not jump up quickly from a chair that is not optimal for you.

If you go somewhere and the chairs don't suit then stand up and walk around. Don't allow other people to dictate that you remain seated and put your back at risk. Stand off to the side or at the back so that you can move unobtrusively and protect your back.

You might think that sitting in chairs is simple because it is something we do all the time and often for many hours a day but it can be the number one thing that it is triggering your back or leg pain. On the book website *www.DrugFreePainReliefBook.com* is a quick bonus video with handy hints.

Another area that can contribute to back and neck pain is your bed or mattress. Do you have to strain to get out of bed? If so, why? Is your mattress too soft? Too old? Deep indentations in which you get stuck? Does it need to be firmer around the edges so you can get out easily? Is it the right height for you to get out without strain or injury?

Do you have a phone in your bedroom? I've lost count of the number of clients that have come to me, having jumped out of bed quickly to grab and answer their phone. Going from a deeply relaxed, horizontal position to an urgent, vertical upright motion does not help pain levels. Perhaps put your phone outside to charge and not have it in the bedroom, or use an alarm clock to wake up in the morning instead. Your priority should be sleep, restoration and for your body to be or remain pain free.

You ultimately have to decide on your priorities. Are you going to be at the beck and call of others to the detriment of you living a life pain free? For example, don't jump up to answer the front door bell, tell them to wait and then take your time. Don't be a slave to your mobile phone. If it's not convenient to answer, then don't! Ring back when it is good for you. The human race has survived without mobile phones for thousands of years, don't let the technology control you.

Make your well-being a priority. If you are injured or in pain, you cannot help anyone else so look after yourself first. Then when you are better, you can assist others. It's similar to the reason they tell you on a plane in an emergency to put your oxygen mask on first, before helping others. Because if you go down, you can't help anyone. Be aware and change your environment to suit you, not the other way around – you are so worth it!

Daily Do's and Don'ts!

If you have pain issues with your upper back or neck:

- When standing or sitting, stop crossing or folding your arms across the front of your body. That position tends to bring your shoulders forward and over time creates a cramped 'round shouldered' posture. Some people like to fold their arms and rest them on their protruding stomachs or breasts but that position is inherently 'lazy', and long term can create a permanently rounded upper back and associated weakness in the thoracic spinal muscles. It can be a bad habit you might like to change if you are serious about becoming pain free in the upper back and neck.

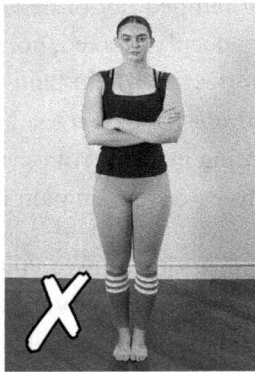

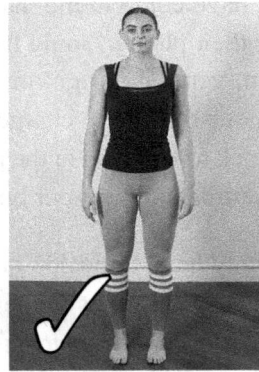

- When sitting, do not clasp your hands together in your lap. As children many of us were taught to do that to keep idle hands still, but now as an adult with pain issues, this may no longer be good for you. If you are sitting upright, your elbows should be hanging relaxed and vertically aligned under your shoulders. Your hands resting gently on your mid upper thighs, allows your shoulders to stay back and for you to have your chest upright and elevated (breathing deeply into the lungs).

- Carrying a heavy handbag repeatedly on one shoulder places enormous pressure on the nerves and muscles and over time can cause imbalances in the upper spine. Use the handle and hold the bag in your hand, changing sides regularly. When carting groceries, evenly distribute the weight in both hands, carry lighter loads and make extra trips if necessary.

> For years I have suffered from migraines, headaches and tension in neck, shoulders and upper back area. Constant headaches are very debilitating and can affect my ability to work. Bowen therapy has really helped give me relief from pain. I am very grateful to get that relief with a treatment that is gentle, non-invasive, inexpensive and it really works.　　　　Serena F.

If you have pain issues with your lower back, hips and knees:

- Do you suffer from iliotibial band (ITB) pain? Pain in the outer thighs? For me personally and for many female clients this can be a real issue. We generally were told as little girls, to be ladies and to always keep our legs together. So we tend to stand with our feet together and also sit in that position.

  However from a body structure point of view, this position can put pressure on the ITB which stretches from your hip to your knee and can create that outer thigh, leg ache. Structurally the body is far more stable when standing with the feet apart. The wider you are in the hips, the further apart your feet may need to be. So simply changing the way you stand over time may help with ITB pain.

- A big stomach and weak core muscles can cause problems such as getting up out of a chair, up off the floor or in and out of the car. Tightening your stomach muscles or engaging your core muscles before putting your back under stress helps protect it from further injury. I had a client who injured her lower back from merely leaning over the bathroom sink to clean her teeth. She had a large stomach and no core muscle tone.

  Whenever you are leaning forward and if you have a big stomach, that extra weight can have a big impact on your pain levels or cause re-injury. Until you regain or develop core strength, you can use your hand to physically support your stomach when leaning forward or temporarily use a back brace.

- If you have back or hip issues, a straight upright chair may be best at least while you're dealing with pain. That way you don't sag into the chair and your spine is upright as possible so you don't have to strain your lower back to get up and get moving.

- Do not cross your legs (standing, sitting or lying) – besides putting pressure on nerve pathways and possibly trigger pain, that position can affect circulation and lymphatic drainage to the lower limbs. It may be an old habit hard to break but if you want to be pain free you need to make the choice!

- Several male clients I have seen, have had a dull or persistent ache in one hip or buttock. Bowen Therapists are aware of 'hip pocket syndrome' where the cause for that type of pain has often been found to come from carrying and sitting on wallets and keys in the back pocket. Those objects in the hip pocket may create a pelvic imbalance when you sit. So consider keeping the back pocket empty. Sitting on your wallet may stop you spending money but in the long run it doesn't help your hip pain!

- When standing, take your weight evenly on both feet. Don't slouch onto one hip or lean to one side. This places huge strain on the pelvis and back. If you are required to stand in one spot for any length of time, keep your body weight evenly distributed and simply bend the back of the knees ever-so slightly. Alternately place your buttocks and back flat against a wall and maintain weight evenly on both feet. If you find this difficult to do, it can be an indication that are structural imbalances and you may benefit from physical correction.

- Walking backwards slowly can sometimes ease lower back pain. Find a safe area where you can walk backwards for up to ten minutes several times a week. Maybe have someone with you to guide and ensure no risk of falls. It puts less strain on your knees and may help correct rotation of the pelvis as well as strengthen supporting muscles. Walking backwards is also challenging and good for the brain.

- When lifting, first move in close to the object, bend your knees, hold your stomach muscles in tight before and as you lift. Do not over reach or twist.

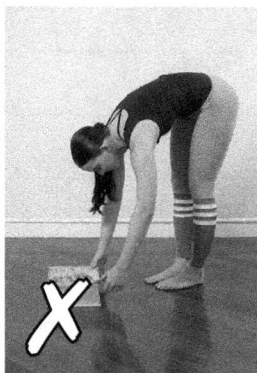

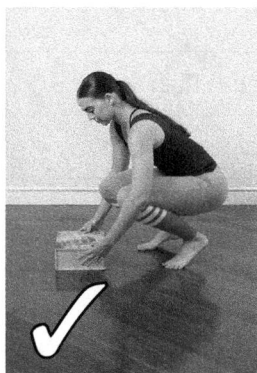

- Entering or alighting from a car. Getting out of a car, most of us tend to 'throw' a leg out and start walking. But if you have lower back or hip pain, you should slow down and think about what you're about to do. To avoid strain on the hips and pelvis, keep knees together, tighten stomach muscles and turn the trunk of your body to the open car doorway.

Depending on the type of car, sit close to the edge of the car seat and swing the legs out together if possible, placing both feet on the ground. You can use your arms to lift your legs if necessary. Try not to get in and out of a car if it is parked on a slope, flat even ground is better for back and leg pain conditions. It might be useful for you to look at the video on the book website for extra tips: *www.DrugFreePainReliefBook.com.*

> *"Become your own body detective! Be aware of your home and work environment. What are you doing that is giving or aggravating your pain?"*
>
> **Suzanne McTier-Browne**

Become aware of how you move. Tune into your body regularly throughout the day and night – how does your body feel? Are there certain activities during the day that trigger or aggravate your pain? Once you are pain free you want to be aware of and avoid anything that can cause re-injury.

Body Detective Questions:
Where exactly is your pain?
Does it change position or is it always in the same place?
Do you have it when you first get up in the morning? If so, what is your rating? No pain I 1 I 2 I 3 I 4 I 5 I 6 I 7 I 8 I 9 I 10 I Most intense pain
Do you have it in the evening or later in the day? If so, what is your rating? No pain I 1 I 2 I 3 I 4 I 5 I 6 I 7 I 8 I 9 I 10 I Most intense pain
When is it worse – in the morning or in the evening?
How frequent is your pain? Is it constant? Is it daily? Is it weekly? Is it monthly? Other?
Does it affect your sleep?
Do you wake up in pain?
Is there an activity or position that makes it worse?
Be really aware of the activities you do today.
Before you do each activity, rate your pain levels. Write it down. After the activity, how are your pain levels? Did they change? Did this activity increase, decrease or made no difference to your pain? If it increased your pain, can you change the activity so it doesn't cause you pain? Or do you really have to do that activity? If it is necessary, can someone else help you or can they do it?

This is a great exercise to see what is actually impacting on your pain levels and with that awareness you can then bring change. If you are in intense pain just doing this for one day will bring some knowledge and insight. Even better if you can manage this for a week to really get an idea of the impact of the things you are doing daily. Respect and love yourself enough to do this little bit of homework.

It will be invaluable in helping you and your health professional identify what is happening in your life that triggers or aggravates your pain. Being a body detective, monitoring my posture and supporting my body as much as possible has helped me stay pain free for more than 30 years.

Suzanne's Squeeze Sequence for a Stiff Neck

Most people have tight muscles in their upper back, neck and shoulders and we've discussed previously how that can easily come about because of working long hours on computers, falling asleep awkwardly or head down using an iPad etc. So if you have a stiff neck and find it hard to turn your head, as a special bonus for readers of this book, I'm sharing a video on my 'simple to use at home' technique. Available at: *DrugFreePainReliefBook.com.*

A Final Comment

I wasn't really sure where to put this case study – 'Sexy Back' (see following page). While it's not strictly about posture, it is about positioning of the body and this client is not the only person that I've seen with this complaint.

Case Study – Sexy Back!

A young female in her early 20s, was having a lot of trouble with her lower back and sciatic nerve. She'd already been hospitalised several times with the pain and there was talk of back surgery but she'd been told to lose weight before that could go ahead. She'd tried other therapies with no relief and then a friend of hers (a client of mine) had told her to see me.

There was structural misalignment in her lower spine and hips – she had grown up on a property and used to ride horses, had several falls, but now worked at an office in the city. She wasn't getting any physical exercise and her muscle tone was very poor. However she responded quickly with her first Bowen session and had significant relief. She was very excited to be able to move with substantially less pain and I spoke to her about needing to rebuild muscle tone to support the corrections, suggested some gentle exercises she could do at home to support her recovery.

Her second session also went well and we got further improvement to the stage where she was no longer in pain. She hadn't however chosen to do any of the exercises or stretches to help herself. I explained again the importance of building and maintaining muscle tone to keep pain free.

Her third treatment was totally different. She came in limping and in severe pain. Her father came in this time with her. She told me she had been great, no pain and full mobility until the weekend, then something had gone drastically wrong – she didn't know what. Her father sat out in reception while I helped his daughter but as I came out of her clinic room he grabbed me.

"She's been going really well coming here but it's her husband." he whispered. "He works away on shifts but he came back over the weekend. A long weekend, it's too much sex or what he makes her do. It's happened before but she won't listen!"

I knew it was possible and could see he was very concerned. Recent activity had made her pelvis unstable and because of her poor muscle tone and lack of fitness she was back in trouble.

So if you are in a similar situation, just be aware of 'sexy back'. There are positions where you can still have fun or a loving connection but not put your back at risk. Slow and supported tends to work better than fast and rough, and honest communication with your partner is important. Be conscious of positions that hurt or trigger your lower back pain and adjust accordingly.

Typically the person with lower back pain would take a more passive role and pillows can be used to support the back, hips or go under the knees, etc. Suggested positions depend on the type of pain and the actions that trigger it but may include seated using a chair or laying on the side and spooning. Having a hot shower before sex can also be helpful and can loosen tight muscles, easing cramp and spasm. Don't hesitate to ask your doctor or therapist for positions specific for your condition – they won't mind, they would rather you use safe positions and stay pain free!

CHAPTER 5

Made to Move
– Move it or Lose it!

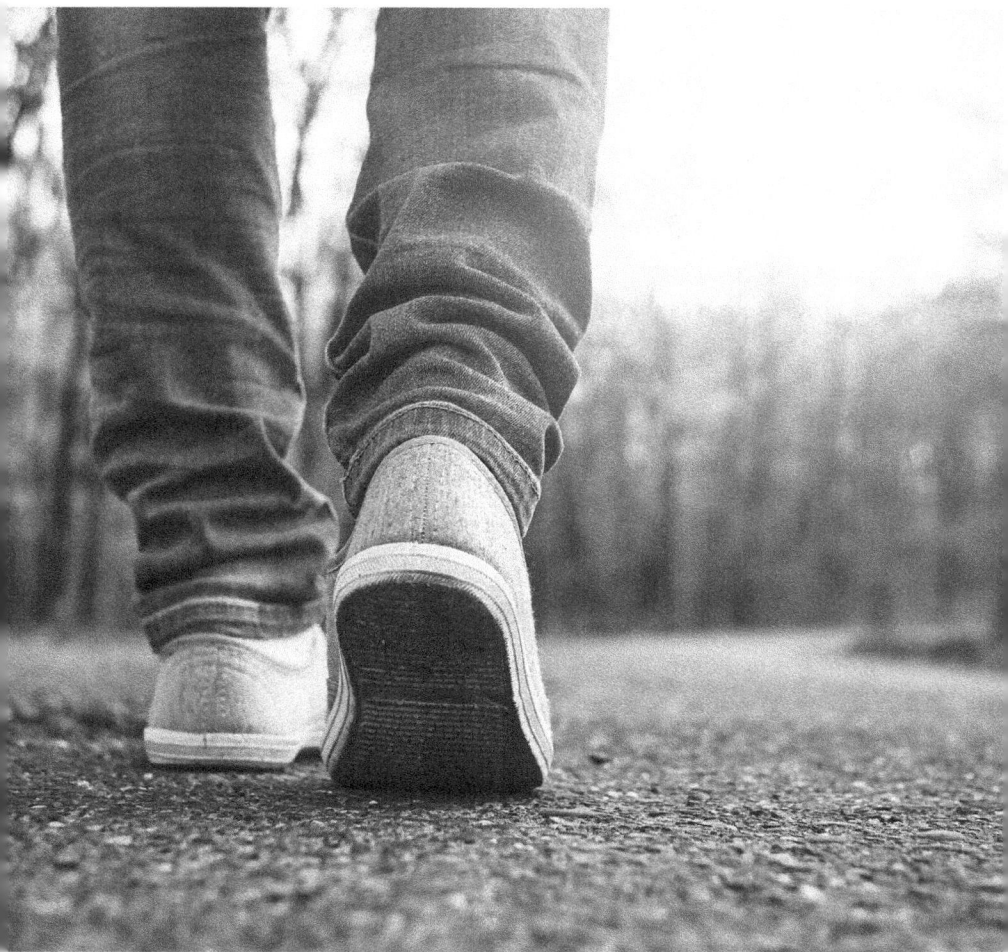

CHAPTER 5

Made to Move
– Move it or Lose it!

"The alternative to daily exercise, stretching or movement is deterioration, aging, loss of muscle tone and circulation, eventually atrophy and the death of healthy tissue – seriously you need to move!"

Suzanne McTier-Browne

When you're hit with that pain and it rocks you to your very core, it seems to bring everything in your life to a screaming halt. If it persists over time, you get worn out and start to care about nothing, including yourself. You may become mentally numb because tuning into your current predicament and processing it is way too painful to bare.

And it's OK to go to ground for a little while. To just go to bed and lick your wounds giving yourself some valuable time to rest, grieve, sleep and just tune it all out, but you cannot stay like that every day. Well actually you can but it serves no positive purpose and doesn't help you long term. Because while you may feel like you're the only person having to deal with this pain, the reality is that people every day are dealing with what you have, and some have it so much worse.

Please remember every day, you have a choice – to do a little something or a big fat nothing. The problem is that staying in bed and doing a 'big fat nothing' also achieves nothing which can quickly become depressing and energy draining. Plus lying around in bed doing nothing for days on end can become quite catastrophic for your body. You lose precious muscle tone that supports your posture and mobility. Once you lose that it takes a lot of work to regain.

Of course it takes far less energy and effort to just give up and have a couple of weeks or months (or years) lost in your own pity party. But then you lose valuable muscle tone and you've just created a massive workload later for yourself. So the easiest way is to maintain what you have during this testing period and then when you are feeling better, build upon it.

> *"If we want to direct our lives, we must take control of our consistent actions. It's not what we do once in a while that shapes our lives, but what we do consistently."*
>
> **Tony Robbins**

When I was fighting my diagnosis, I realised that movement was crucial and because of its fast progression, I also knew that I didn't have the luxury to lie in bed feeling sorry for myself. I was terrified of being confined to a wheelchair and knew that if I gave up and didn't move, that my demise would come so much faster. So even though I was in immense pain, I decided I would walk as much as possible or swim when the pressure and pain in my joints was too much to bare.

This was in the day before gyms and personal training were in fashion and so I devised exercise programs for myself. Simple worked really well because while I was motivated, I tired so easily. If I tried to do too much too soon I would get frustrated, then depressed and very tempted to give up. So I knew I had to step up, take responsibility and control my attitude and outlook.

I set myself small achievable goals every day and started with just a simple walk around the house. We lived in a double-storey house so even getting up and down the stairs was a huge effort. So many times I slowly crawled up the stairs on my hands and knees or came down on my bottom. But I was determined not to be stuck in my bedroom and nothing was going to stop me.

Around this time, the improvements from having corrective bodywork were really starting to show and I was able to start doing more. I couldn't drive at that stage even though I had a car, so I pulled out my old high school bicycle and started to take short rides as I desperately needed a change of scenery. At that point my coordination and steering wasn't the best but I just rode in the quiet streets around my house and I felt such a sense of achievement.

No one coached or trained me, I had to be determined and self-motivated. So how much do you want to become pain free? Even if you are lacking resources or support, it doesn't matter! Just dig deep, take action and do something, anything!

> *"Even in the depths of your pain, life is all about choices. You can choose to fight and take action, and you can do it by yourself or with a support team."*
>
> **Suzanne McTier-Browne**

The thing is, as humans we are part of the animal kingdom and are made to move – in all directions, every day. Seeing a structural therapist to correct your posture and body alignment should make movement, stretching and exercise easier for you.

We were not designed to sit all day at a computer desk, be in a car driving around for hours or working a 12-hour shift in a mining truck etc. We are biped with long legs and arms for a reason – we are made to walk, run, jog, dance, stretch, climb and reach.

Our anatomy and physiology is such that if we don't constantly move, our muscles and joints do physically become stiff and our fascia (connective tissue or membranes that surround our muscles, stabilises our bodies etc.) will actually start to fuse together and then limit our mobility.

Dr Gil Hedley, in his 'The Fuzz Speech' video on YouTube illustrates this attribute of fascia so well. He shows a normal moving joint versus one that is immobile and has built up so much 'fuzz' that it has 'frozen' into place. (Warning, the video takes place in an autopsy lab and does show human remains – thank you to those who donate their bodies to science so that we all can learn.) From Dr Hedley's video:

> *One of the great benefits of bodywork whether it be massage or structural therapies or physical therapy or any kind of hands on therapy, these types of therapies introduce movement manually to tissues that have become fuzzed over through lack of movement whether the lack of movement is because of an injury and a person is protecting that injury or because of a personality expression ... so you can grow fuzz by choice or by accident ... you can take responsibility for melting the fuzz and if there is too much fuzz in your body and it's frozen up you might like to seek help in order to introduce movement.*

So if your chronic pain has meant that movement is restricted or difficult and you haven't done so in a while, you may need some help to get started. Actually most successful people (in any field) use some kind of support team to help them and then stay in peak condition, so don't think you've failed if you need help.

> I had extreme pain in my right neck and shoulder. About two weeks before seeking Bowen Therapy, I was unable to sleep or sit for any period. Spent majority of my time standing to try and prevent pain, not able to use my arm at work. Since successful treatment, am sleeping a lot better. I am able to sit and relax now before and after work. I have little to no pain after three treatments with Suzanne. I am also able to go back to playing sport and exercising every day without constant aching or lack of movement in my neck and shoulder.   Donna S.

Hopefully by now, you've found yourself a talented therapist who is helping you with your posture and body structural corrections, improving your circulation, lymphatic drainage and mobility. You can also choose someone to assist with your movement program or do it yourself. You are in control.

Your support team may consist of any of the following:

- Your Doctor, Naturopath or Homeopath

- Physical therapists eg Bowen Therapist, Reflexologist, Massage Therapist or Chiropractor

- Exercise or stretch specialists, eg. Physiotherapist, Exercise Physiologist, Yoga Teacher or Personal Trainer

Find a fun sport or activity you enjoy once you are moving more freely. If you have deterioration in your bones or joints, low impact is generally the way to go so walking, swimming, water aerobics, yoga, tai chi, dancing and gym could be good options. Just an extra comment regarding pool exercise. I've had several clients who had accidents getting in and out, slipping on wet floors and ladders, so please be careful.

Of course, not everyone lives in a large city with easy access to expertise and equipment, so the following home stretches and exercises have been provided for general information. Please note, I am not an exercise specialist however as a therapist I know the basics and during the past 30 years of getting myself pain free and staying that way, I have tried many. Also in clinic, I've found particular stretches which work well for many people.

However everyone is unique with different abilities and health conditions so you have the control and responsibility to select what is appropriate for you in your current situation, or check with your doctor or health professional. It is not expected that you will do all the stretches and exercises in this book, but choose the relevant and helpful ones for you.

You may have had pain for only for a short period and still be able to do most activities. If you find the following too easy then you may decide to commence advanced activities or sport. Alternatively if you have been battling pain for a long time, you may have greatly reduced fitness and muscle tone from inactivity. Only you know.

Some tips before you start any movement program:

✓ **Move with intention** – don't be in a rush. First stop and think what you want to achieve. Secondly visualise it clearly in your mind, mentally feel yourself doing it successfully and then finally make your move. Be deliberate and thoughtful in your actions and you greatly increase success. You also will decrease your chance of accident or injury.

✓ **Do any new activity slowly.** If you been in pain for a while, chances are you've lost some muscle tone and flexibility due to inactivity. Suddenly calling those weakened muscles and joints into fast action is not in your best interest. Start slowly!

✓ **Protect your lower back.** Statistically the majority of people experience their pain in the lower back, hips and legs. One of the most important things you can do to protect yourself is to tighten your stomach muscles, engage your core, before and whenever you put your back under strain, particularly if you are overweight or have a large stomach. For example, when getting in and out of chairs or your car, lifting groceries out of the car boot etc, pull in and tighten those stomach muscles before and during the activity. This will help support the lower back and reduce the potential for injury.

✓ **Start in small ways** – with your everyday activities. Go for a short walk first thing in the morning or in the evening rather than watching TV. Take the dog for a walk (or your partner, children or grandchildren). Take every opportunity to move rather than staying in bed or in that chair! That old saying is true, 'move it or lose it!' Start with small, realistic goals and work your way up gradually.

✓ **Get out of the house!** A change of location can increase your energy levels, allow interaction with people, create a diversion and take the focus off your pain. A walk in the garden, along the river or at the beach can give you fresh air to breathe and help improve morale. If you are alone, head to your nearest shopping centre or park and make some new friends.

✓ **Adopt a positive 'YES' attitude.** Whenever you get invited anywhere, automatically say yes! Even if you don't feel like it, the majority of times when you make the effort and get there, you will be glad you did and your body will appreciate the variety of activity and movement.

✓ **Get out of your pyjamas!** When you are not feeling well, you're tired and you could just stay in bed all day, please don't! It's so easy to get stuck in that rut and then the days drag into weeks and months and you just get weaker and weaker. If the least you do in a day is to drag yourself out of bed, clean your teeth, get dressed and brush your hair – you've done well. Give yourself a simple daily "must do" routine and commit to looking after yourself!

> *"Small purposeful steps consistently over time makes for big improvements in your health and relieving your pain!"*
>
> **Suzanne McTier-Browne**

I had arthritis in my knee after having the kneecap removed. Excruciating pain for eight very long weeks. Unable to walk without massive doses of painkillers. Have had three Bowen treatments and pain almost gone. A few niggles now and again and a bit stiff but no excruciating pain. My whole body feels better! Thanks Suzanne, thought I was never going to feel pain free again. Would highly recommend it to anyone and I do frequently. Marion M.

(Shortly after Marion gave this testimonial and had her fourth Bowen, she became pain free. She regained full mobility and was able to start regularly exercising which greatly improved her quality of life.)

If your pain has kept you sedentary, then any movement is valuable. Even if you are chair bound there will still be parts of your body you can move. If you can't move yourself, get someone to assist you. Moving and stretching usually feels good, sometimes initially there is a little discomfort but never stretch into pain. Treat yourself with love and respect and most importantly don't give up, your goal is to keep moving. There are so many benefits:

✓ improves your cardiac health, gets your heart pumping and improves circulation

✓ improves your breathing and lung function

✓ strengthens your muscles and joints and helps with balance and preventing falls

✓ improves flexibility, movement and will enable you to do everyday tasks more easily

✓ helps maintain bone density

✓ increased blood and lymphatic flow helps improve skin elasticity and healing

✓ helps you feel better, relieves stress and you will feel a sense of accomplishment

✓ you will look and feel younger with increased energy and stamina

Also protect yourself if you are getting help with your stretches and exercises – do not allow anyone to test or push you into pain. Numerous clients have come to clinic because they have over-stretched, hurt themselves in a too vigorous exercise routine or their pain has been inflamed in the process of being tested and diagnosed. You need to be honest with your health professionals and let them know when something is increasing your pain.

So the truth is that a movement program takes effort and commitment, however the benefits are immeasurable and the alternative is very scary.

Getting started may not be easy but you just have to do it if you want to relieve your pain long term.

> *"You can't afford to be lazy or blasé with your health. Your body is your most precious asset so your priority, time and care should be invested in supporting and maintaining where you live."*
>
> **Suzanne McTier-Browne**

Lower Back Stretches

The following stretches may assist you with releasing tight muscles, improving flexibility and circulation in the back and legs which can then allow pressure to come off nerve pathways and pain levels to decrease.

If you have difficulty getting down and up off the floor, make sure you have a stool or chair (not on wheels) to assist you or someone nearby. When lying on the floor, you may need to cushion your spine by lying on a yoga mat or carpet. If needed you can use a small pillow or towel to support your head. If mobility is an issue, some of these stretches can be done on a firm bed or in a chair.

Remember you have the choice and the power – you are also responsible for your recovery so use common sense and do not stretch into pain. When you are dealing with chronic pain, you have to be respectful and patient with your body, your recovery may take some time and that is OK. If you need help be responsible enough to ask for it, don't put yourself at risk. Your goal is to improve your situation, not to get angry, frustrated or injure yourself.

Starting out you might only be able to do one or two repetitions of a stretch, that's fine. If you do these daily or even every second or third day, you'll gradually build up to more repetitions and then you'll be ready to move onto a more advanced movement program.

Remember to do these exercises and stretches slowly and focused. Don't rush between them or to change positions. Stop between each one, visualise in your head what you want to do and then picture yourself successfully achieving it. Once you have that image clear in your mind then go ahead and complete it.

Devoting full attention means no mobile phones or doing this while watching TV, etc. You want full focus on your body and what you are doing. Many people were injured initially by not being mindful or concentrating on what they were doing.

> *"Move mindfully and with intent – where the mind goes first, the body will follow more easily."*
>
> **Suzanne McTier-Browne**

Breathe deeply as much as possible during these exercises. Belly or diaphragmatic breathing helps take your body out of 'stress' mode and will help you relax. Holding your breath too long may raise blood pressure.

Don't do stretches cold. Warm up first by walking on the spot or doing gentle movement, having a warm shower or applying a heat pack on the problem area.

The following stretches and exercises are not for acute pain, recent accident or injury. See your doctor or health professional for advice in those cases. You can come back to these activities once you have moved past the emergency phase. And remember you do not have to do all of the following, choose which are relevant for you.

Floor (on Elbows):

This gentle position can be a good way to start helping yourself at home.

- Lie flat on the floor on your stomach and relax your back. Once this position is comfortable, come up to lean and rest on your elbows (ideally directly under the shoulders). Relax in that position for a couple of minutes depending on your pain level. If resting on your elbows is too high at this stage, come down and rest your chin onto your hands.
- You can do this position several times during the day if you wish.
- To get up off the floor, consider tightening the stomach muscles to protect your lower back and move slowly.

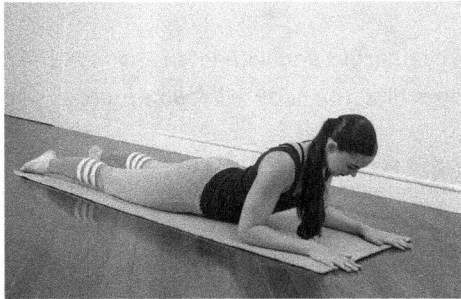

Feet on Chair:

- Lie on your back on the floor and place your feet up onto a chair. Relax for up to ten minutes.
- Focus on breathing deeply and you have the option of slowly turning your head to one side, then the other, coming back to centre before relaxing.
- Hand option: palms up can help to open up the chest, shoulders and start to reverse round shouldered posture.

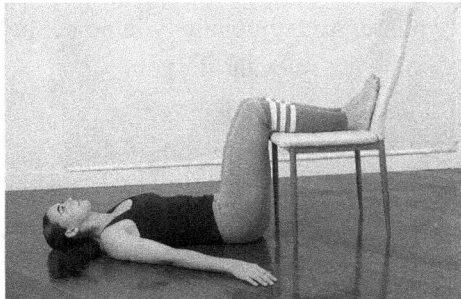

Floor Stretch:

- Lie on your back on the floor and gently stretch your arms above your head, breathing deeply.
- Stretch and elongate the body, from finger tips to toes.
- Slowly point and then flex the toes, gently relax.

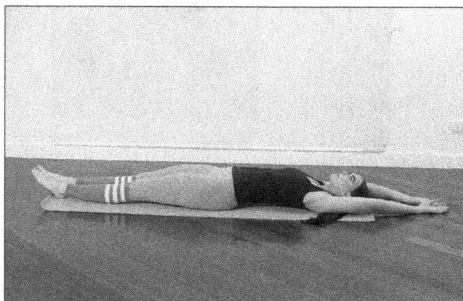

Pelvic Tilts:

- Lie on your back, knees bent and feet flat on the floor.
- Stomach muscles tightened, gently curl your tailbone up and towards you, your lower back will tend to flatten on the floor. Hold for several seconds.
- Slowly lower your tailbone back to the floor and your spine to naturally curve.
- Continue for three to ten repetitions. These are small movements, gently rocking the tailbone.

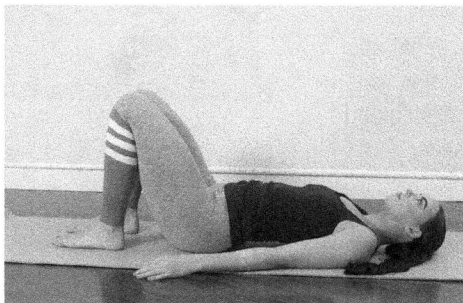

Knee to Chest:

- Lie on your back on the floor and slowly bend your knees placing your feet flat on the floor. Adjust your hips and lower back so you feel comfortable.

- Gently stretch and lengthen your spine (from tailbone to the crown of your head) chin should be in a natural and neutral position.

- Bend one knee up to your chest and grab your knee/leg with two hands if possible. If that is too hard use a belt or towel. Hold the stretch as long as comfortable and then slowly release down onto the floor. When you start you may only be able to do the stretch for a couple of seconds, that's OK. Remember to keep breathing.

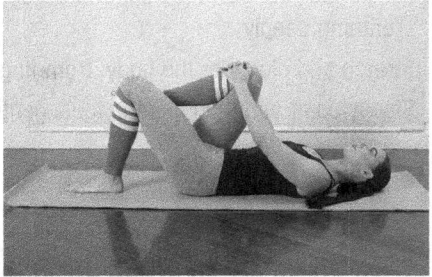

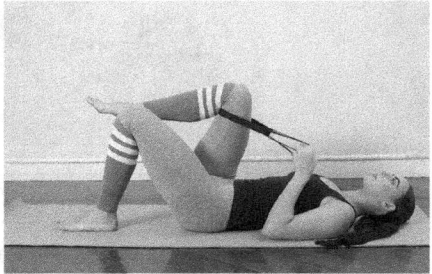

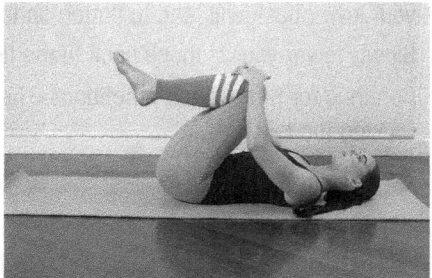

- Bend the other knee towards your chest and repeat as above. If comfortable, you can repeat the stretch and alternate the knees.

- Option: you can also do this stretch with both knees together and hugging them into your chest.

- Option: if lower back or hip pain is not an issue, the resting or non-stretched leg can be fully extended to lie flat on the floor while the bent knee is brought to chest.

Lying Hamstring Stretch:

- Lie on your back, slowly bend your knees and place both feet flat on the floor. Adjust your hips and back for comfort.

- Bring one knee up towards your chest and grasp it with both hands Slowly extend and straighten the knee so you can feel the stretch into the back of the leg. Hold your leg at the back of your thigh or you can use a band, belt or towel and hook it around the ball of your foot. Hold for 10–30 seconds. You can also flex the ankle slowly up and down while holding this position. Don't forget to breathe!

- When you are ready to lower the leg, gently bend the knee first and then lower the leg to the floor.

- Repeat stretch with the other leg.

- Option: if it is too hard to get down onto the floor, you can do this seated in a chair or standing with foot elevated on a step.

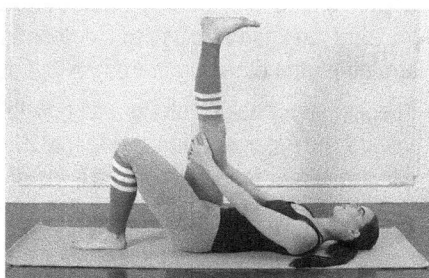

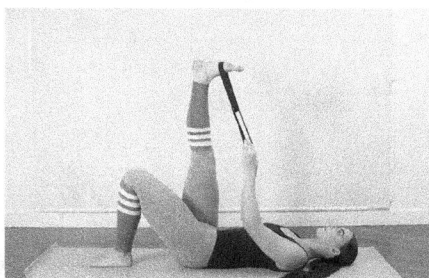

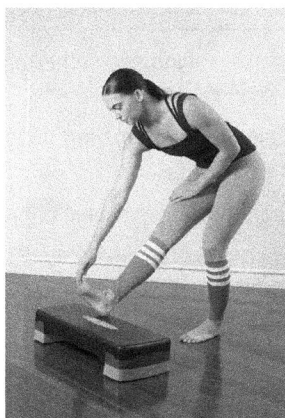

Seated Hamstring Stretch:

- Seated on the floor, bend one knee and bring that foot near your body, keeping the knee as close to the floor as you can comfortably. Extend and straighten the other leg in front of you, foot flexed and toes up to the ceiling.
- Keeping your back as straight as possible, lean forward at the hips and toward the outstretched leg and foot. Use a band, belt or towel around the ball of the foot to hold the stretch (pointing the toes, lessens the stretch).
- Repeat stretch with the other leg.
- Sitting on a cushion or block to raise the hips may help with this stretch.

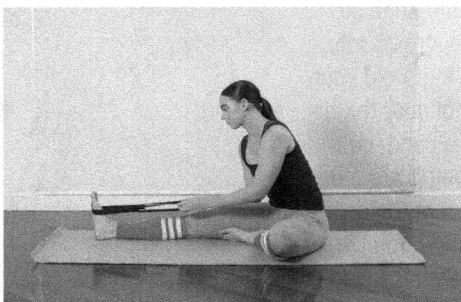

Floor Groin Stretch:

- Sit with feet facing each other and together, knees bent and comfortably low to the floor.
- The closer your feet to your body the more intense the stretch but work within your limits.
- Sitting on a cushion or block to raise the hips may help with this stretch.
- Option: can be done standing. Legs apart, bend one knee and lean to the side, to feel stretch in the other hip and groin.

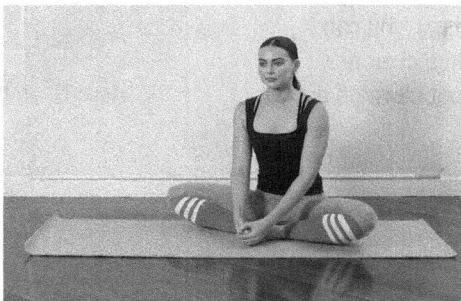

Calf Stretch:

- May also assist with cramping and tight ankles.
- Standing a short distance away from a wall, gently lean forward and push against it with the leg you want to stretch behind you.
- Keep your heel of that back leg planted to the floor or as close as you can. You can adjust the angle of your foot by leaning further into the wall. The greater the angle of your ankle and foot, the more it stretches the lower leg.

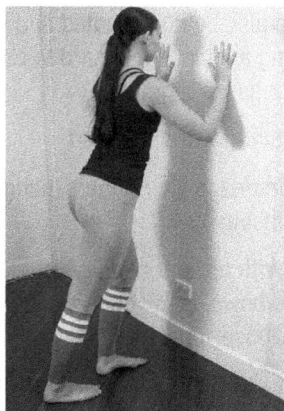

Neck, Shoulder & Chest Stretches

As discussed in Chapter Four, with the overuse of computers, mobile phones, iPads, computer games, etc., many of us spend a lot of time with our heads tilted forward, sitting for long periods in poor posture with rounded shoulders and spine. This sets us up for pain, tight muscles and being prone to neck and shoulder injury. The following may help stretch and relax your muscles, relieve tightness due to that poor posture and even if you do not have pain, these may be good for prevention and maintenance.

Again be present and listen to your body. Stretch and lengthen the spine by stretching from the tailbone to the crown of the head and keep your rib cage lifted off the hips where possible. Breathe deeply and relax as you do these activities. The neck stretches can generally be done seated or standing.

Head forward (or down onto chest) exercises are not included as I've found many clients with headaches, migraines and neck issues do not benefit and can have their symptoms worsen. However everyone is unique and your doctor or exercise specialist may prescribe such exercises for you.

Standing Overhead Stretch:

Can also be done seated and using a towel if it is hard to clasp your hands together.

- Stand with feet apart.

- Interlace your fingers, palms facing out.

- With a slight bend in your elbows, take your arms up above your head, inhale.

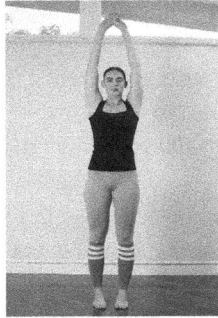
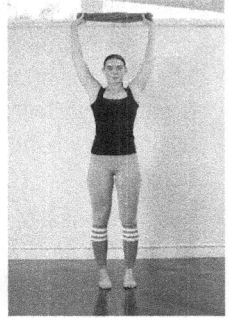

- Exhale, stretch your arms and press your palms upwards.

- Keep breathing. When ready to release, exhale and gently lower the arms down.

Side Stretch:

Can also be done seated and using a towel if it is hard to clasp your hands together.

- Stand with feet apart.

- Inhale and take your arms up above your head.

- Either clasp your fingers together or hold the wrist of one arm with the other hand.

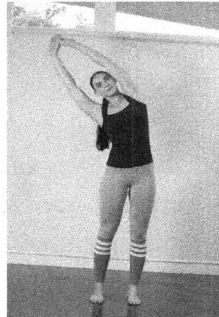

- Exhale and gently lean to one side (this will create a stretch in the opposite side).

- Keep breathing. When ready to release, exhale, gently come back to centre and then lower the arms down.

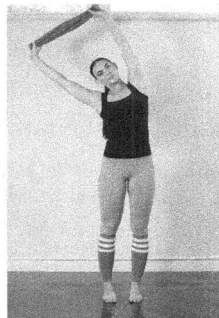

- Repeat leaning to the opposite side.

Side Neck Turns:

Can be done seated or standing. If you have a sore neck, turn to the better side first.

- Relax, release and lower your shoulders, your head facing to the front.

- Slowly turn your head to one side towards the shoulder to your comfort level.

- Hold for three to ten seconds, and then slowly come back to centre. Repeat sequence with the other side.

- Ideally do this sequence at least three times.

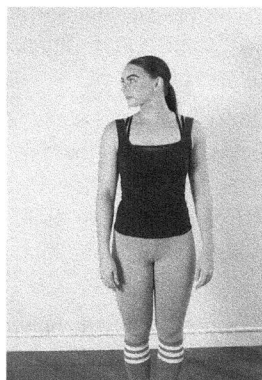

Tilted Neck Stretch:

Can be done seated or standing.

- Relax, release and lower your shoulders, your head facing to the front. Inhale.

- After exhalation, stretch your neck gently upwards through the back or crown of the head. Keep breathing.

- After exhalation, tilt your neck to one side, ear towards the shoulder. Make sure the head does not fall forward.

- Comfortably hold that position for 10–30 seconds, keep breathing and feel the muscles gently stretch on opposite side.

- Do not come out of the stretch quickly. After exhalation, slowly return your head to the middle upright position. If needed, you can use your hand to support or gently start your head moving back to centre.

- Repeat with the other side.

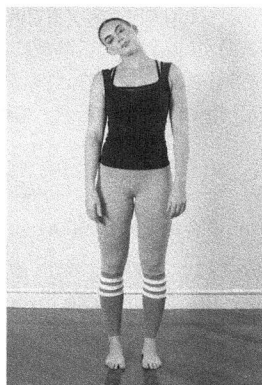

Basic Chest Stretch:

- Stand with your hands on your hips, standing tall with shoulders relaxed and down.
- Slowly bring your shoulders back and your elbows towards each other, this will create a gentle stretch in the chest. Hold for 10–30 seconds and then slowly release.
- Option: clasp hands behind your back and squeeze shoulder blades together.
- Option: hands up, upper arms approximately horizontal to your shoulders. Squeeze your shoulder blades together in the upper back, hold for 10–30 seconds. Feel the stretch into the chest and front of shoulders. Can also be done against a wall.

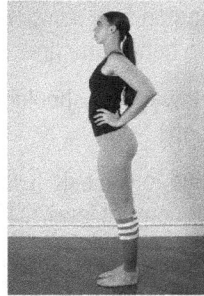

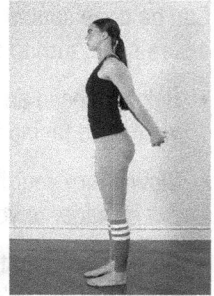

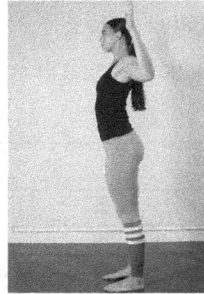

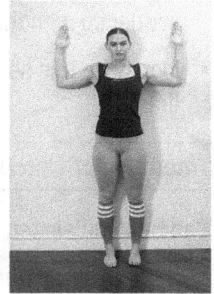

Doorway Chest Stretch:

- Stand in an open doorway.
- Reach up, holding onto top of door frame and lean forward slightly until feeling a gentle stretch in front of chest. Do not overbalance or fall through the doorway.
- Option: if the doorway is too high, reach off to the sides of the door frame as high as you can comfortably reach.
- Release and gently bring arms down.
- Take arms horizontally to the nine and three o'clock positions.
- Lean forward slightly until feeling a gentle stretch in front of chest.
- Wall option: place your hands up and outstretched onto a wall and lean in. Squeeze shoulder blades together and feel a stretch into the chest.

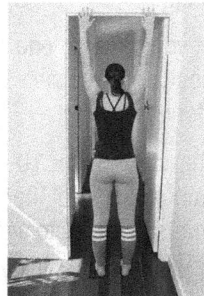

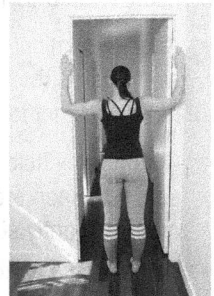

Tricep Stretch:

- Stand feet apart.
- Taking arms up, grab the elbow on one side and gently stretch it up and towards the back. Keep neck and shoulder relaxed as possible.
- Reach your fingertips down between the shoulder blades.
- Relax and breathe deeply.
- For extra stretch, gently lift the chest.
- Come out of the stretch slowly and then do the opposite side.

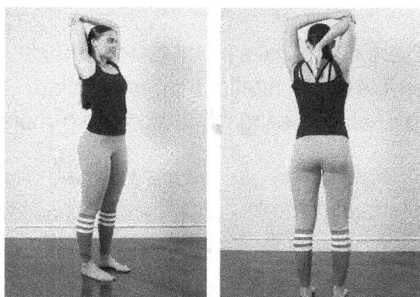

Shoulder Rotations

Because modern day posture tends to be over-developed in a forward position, most people need more backward rotations to help reverse. Can also be done seated.

- Stand with feet apart.
- Stretch and lengthen through the spine (pull up through the back or crown of the head).
- Lift your shoulders gently up and then rotate backwards and bring shoulders down. Repeat and rotate backward up to ten times, then relax.
- Option: Place your finger tips on your shoulders. Bring elbows together in front where comfortable, move up to ceiling, then roll back as far as possible and then down. You should feel the movement in the upper back and the shoulder blades.

Go to

DrugFreePainReliefBook.com

for a free instructional video on arm and shoulder rotations.

Foot Massage

There are reflexes in the feet that relate to the rest of the body. Many people get pain relief from releasing the feet. If you can't get a professional reflexology treatment, you can help yourself by working your own feet.

Sit comfortably and roll a massage ball under the foot, to allow the muscles and tendons to flex and stretch. You can also concentrate on certain areas of the foot for different parts of the body:

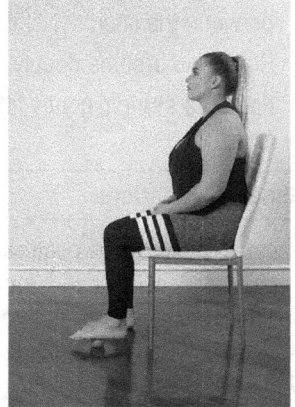

- Head and neck – the toes

- Chest – the ball of the foot

- Spine and back – along the inside or arch of the foot from heel to big toe

- Stomach and bowel – middle of foot, in the arch.

The human foot was designed to walk on natural surfaces such as grass, sand and soil with undulations and natural cushioning. Our feet were not meant to stand all day and walk on hard surfaces such as concrete, tiles and bitumen.

Wearing shoes all the time, also stops the foot from flexing, stretching and adapting to the environment so muscles become stiff and underutilised. Rolling a massage or tennis ball under the arch of the foot helps release and flex those muscles and improve circulation. Wriggle those toes, stretch and flex the feet, rotate the ankles in both directions.

Look after and maintain your feet. See a Reflexologist or Bowen Therapist for professional help if you have issues. Regularly have a pedicure or do your own to exfoliate the layers of dead skin, trim nails and attend to calluses and corns. Some deformities in the feet come from neglect and can change the way you walk, causing further problems with ankles, knees, hips and back. Looking after your feet helps keep you pain free!

Suzanne's Super Seven

Here's my easy exercise routine to get the body moving first thing in the morning. The following generally help with mobility, circulation, lymphatic drainage and work the major muscle groups. They can be also done in the evening before bed to help release tension. You don't have to do all seven, you should select the right exercises for you or ask your doctor or exercise professional. It is recommended that you watch the bonus instructional video on the Super Seven at *www.DrugFreePainReliefBook.com* before starting.

1. Marching on the Spot: Start low impact, gently marching on the spot. It's up to you how long and fast you march and how high you raise your feet. This can also be done between each exercise to keep moving.
2. Breathe and Shake: Stand with feet approximately hip width apart and knees slightly bent. Deep breathe in and stretch your hands and arms up to the sky.   As you exhale, shake your hands above your head and then continue shaking them all the way down to your sides. Let your neck, shoulders, hips and knees gently move and shake as they want. Do at least three times. Wonderful for your circulation and lymphatic system.
3. Side Steps: Start with small steps first to one side, then the other. As you warm up and get more fit you can make those steps bigger. When stronger and used to this activity, you may decide to bend your knees as you step out to the sides and use your arms.
4. Arm Swing: Feet shoulder width apart, shoulders relaxed and arms loosely by your side. Tighten your core or stomach muscles.   Slowly turn to one side and let your arms flop and follow, then slowly turn to the other side. Gradually increase your speed of turning from side to side, letting the arms move and stay loose.
5. Shoulder Rotations and Side Neck Turns: As discussed earlier in this chapter.

6. Air punches:

Standing balanced with feet apart, hands held up and closed into fists, punch upwards into the air above your head with one arm. Bring back to centre and then alternate with the other arm.

You can also lower the arms and air punch directly to the front. May also help to relieve stress and over time extend the range of movement in the shoulders.

7. Air Squats or Chair Sit:

Stand with your feet hip width apart, toes pointing slightly outward and tighten your stomach or core muscles. With a comfortably straight back and upright torso, your weight balanced on your heels, bend at the hips pushing your buttocks backwards and bending the knees like you are about to sit down. Lower to a comfortable and safe level for you, keeping your hips above knee level. Your knees over but not beyond your toes. Return slowly to your starting position.

If this is a new exercise for you, don't go too deep too soon. Place a chair behind you and sit or squat down onto it. After practice, aim to sit down and get up without using your arms, just the strength in your legs, hips and knees. Do squats slowly to your comfort level and build up the number gradually. If there is any discomfort, stop and seek professional guidance.

Final Word on Stretches and Exercise

It can be frustrating when you can't do the things you used to. You may have been fighting this pain battle a long time and you may have had setbacks. Sometimes life is totally unfair – but you can't change the past. The more you relive what happened to you, the more you get trapped in a negative and unproductive cycle that makes you miserable and probably a unpleasant person to be around.

If you can't be bothered to move, stretch and exercise for yourself, then maybe consider your family and friends. When you refuse to change and choose to stay angry and bitter you impact on them also. So step up and take responsibility for your recovery – you are stronger than you think. With a bit of work and commitment you could become a shining example for those around you – wouldn't that be amazing?

CHAPTER 6

What You Put in Your Mouth Counts!

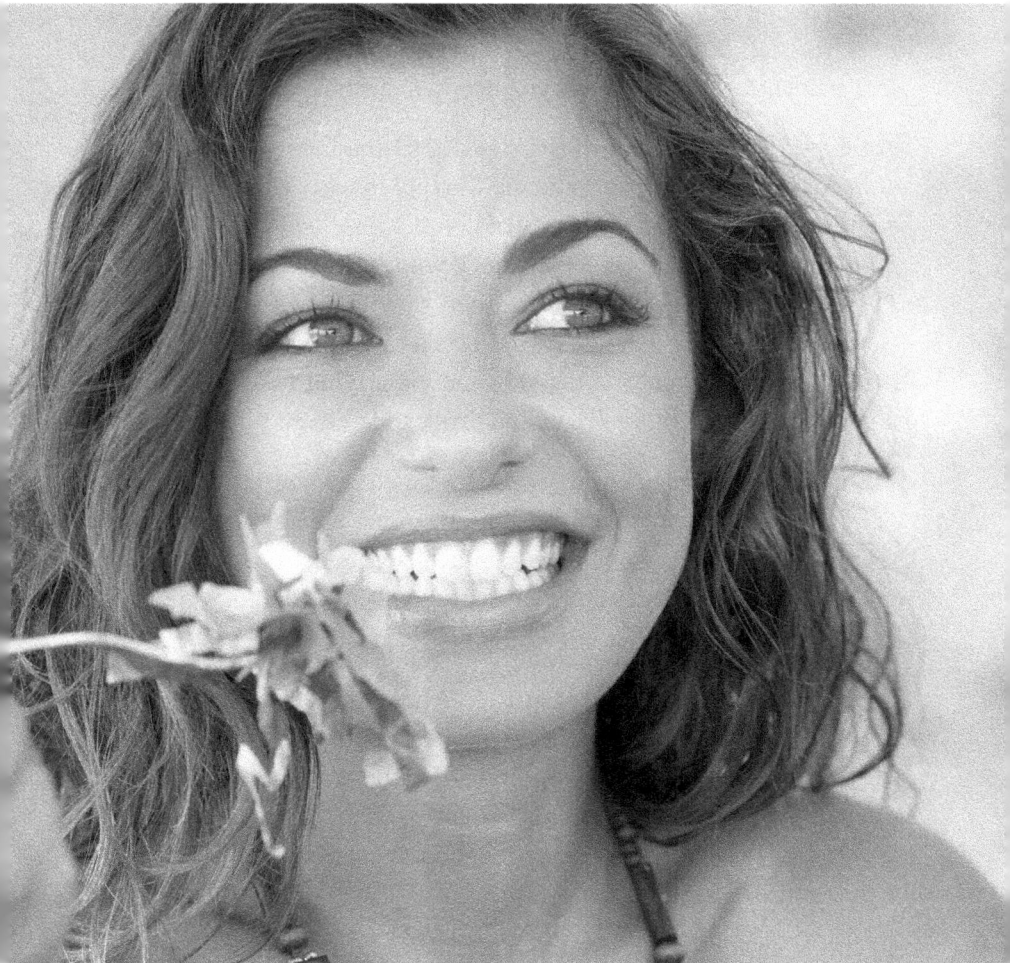

CHAPTER 6

What You Put in Your Mouth Counts!

There are often multiple factors to consider in resolving pain long term. If your pain experience is less than three months (acute) and you are in good physical condition, eat healthily and are young (in age or outlook), you may only need quality bodywork and to monitor your posture to become pain free and stay that way. But if you are in poor health or haven't looked after yourself (be honest), then you have to be realistic and acknowledge that there may be some areas you need to change and improve.

An experienced health professional can see and feel a real difference in skin colour and texture in someone who is active and eats healthily versus someone who consumes only "dead" food, little water and is inactive. It is so much easier to work on someone who looks after themselves. There is more pliability in the muscles and they respond well to treatment. Someone who is dehydrated and/or eats lots of 'dead' food can have little movement or resilience in the skin and underlying tissues and that is not a good thing, remember stagnation can lead to death!

Fresh fruit and vegetables that are consumed raw are 'alive' because the life force of the plant largely remains and important nutrients and enzymes are mostly retained which then help heal and benefit the body. However over cooking and processing can easily turn 'live' food into 'dead' food.

Referring back to the car analogy, we wouldn't expect our cars to perform well on poor quality or inappropriate fuel. We need to respect ourselves as much as a beloved car – hopefully more! Food is the body's fuel and it is very difficult to operate at your best if the fuel you are consuming is low quality or contaminated. Rubbish in equals rubbish out, particularly if we are dealing with pain because poor food choices can have real and long term painful consequences.

Living Food

Fresh 'live' food has the ability to restore life and vitality as it provides the essential energy and building blocks for the body to live, move and repair itself. So consuming living foods such as fresh fruit and vegetables is a big part of relieving your pain.

As well as natural high quality vitamins and minerals that your body can readily utilise, there are valuable enzymes and cofactors that are just not obtainable from cooked or highly processed foods. A large part of your diet should come from raw and living foods if you are serious about getting rid of your pain.

I'm not saying that you should not eat meat – good protein is essential – but I have noticed in clinic that many people with chronic pain conditions eat little fresh food. Most of the foods they consume are cooked. Introducing salads, fresh vegetable juices and fruits can really speed up healing and pain relief.

Chewing and Pooing!

Ok, maybe not the best headline but hopefully it gets your attention about two really important but often neglected points. You could be buying and preparing the best food but if you are not chewing it properly then you are losing a lot of the nutritional benefit. Digestion or pre-digestion actually starts in the mouth.

Chewing is supposed to mechanically breakdown the food into small enough particles so that there is enough surface area for it to mix thoroughly with saliva and enzymes in the mouth for the digestion of starch. If you just take one bite and then swallow quickly, pre-digestion does not happen effectively.

Particles too large in size and which didn't adequately go through that first process, land in the stomach which will struggle to further process and digest (proteins). That liquid, called chyme, then moves to the duodenum where pancreatic enzymes and liver bile mix before passing into the small intestines where the majority of nutrients are absorbed into the body. After that process, the large intestine or colon reabsorbs water and minerals back into the body and the remaining waste matter then goes on to be excreted during defecation.

So have you ever been to the toilet, done your business and then noticed bits of identifiable food floating in the toilet bowl, eg. corn etc? If you had chewed your food properly in the first place that shouldn't happen. This means the nutrients that were stored in those bits of food were not released and made available to your body, it really is waste! Some points to note:

- Chew your food thoroughly, until it is fully mixed with saliva and is liquid in your mouth.

- Don't wash half-chewed food down with water, alcohol or coffee. This also means you probably haven't chewed enough and that extra unnecessary liquid can dilute digestion in the stomach.

- Save your drinking for at least half an hour before or after eating.

- Be focused and relaxed when you eat. Don't multitask as you'll be more likely to swallow without chewing. Also eating while stressed can negatively affect your digestion.

- If your digestion is poor, you may benefit from taking apple cider vinegar before your meal (maybe a teaspoon in a small amount of water or honey). Digestive enzymes may also be beneficial.

So let's further discuss the end of the digestion process – excretion, defecation, poo! It's important no matter how you refer to it. If we think of your body like a house – it's where you live. Do you take out your rubbish or garbage every day? You should but even if you don't, you would understand the importance of why.

Living with garbage increases exposure to germs, bacteria and the risk of illness or disease. The longer you leave it, the more it decomposes and smells. Pests are attracted to garbage so we don't want to leave it in our house and ideally it should be disposed of every day.

A very similar thing happens with the garbage or waste in our bodies. However, there is one really important difference. Our colon is so effective at reabsorbing water and minerals from waste that if we allow that 'garbage' to sit there for more than a day or so, it will continue to do its thing. The faeces will start to dry out and harden and then it becomes more difficult to eliminate and excrete.

Unfortunately as well as absorbing that extra water, toxins can also be reabsorbed back into the body. As well as becoming constipated, you can become toxic and this can increase pain levels. It is in your best interest to keep things moving every day!

✓ Get lots of good fibre from fresh fruits and vegetables.

✓ Drink lots of good water.

✓ Empty the garbage at least every day. If you are eating fresh, healthy food, you will ideally go two or three times a day.

✓ Some medications increase constipation, so check with your doctor or pharmacist as to whether you will need extra assistance.

✓ If you need help to get things moving, do it. Don't hang onto that waste!

Case Study – Being Bullied

A 10-year-old girl came for assistance with back and leg pain plus anxiety. She was being bullied at school because of her excess weight and this, plus her lack of physical exercise and poor diet, were all contributing to her anxiety and sadness. At the first session, it quickly became apparent that the real issue was poor parenting decisions.

There was an obvious weight issue which was contributing to her physical aches and pains, and so the tactful question was – what did my client eat? Her mother replied that because her daughter had once got food poisoning (a couple of years ago) from eating a salad (they think), it had been decided that she would not eat salad or vegetables anymore.

My young client declared she would only eat hamburgers and chips or cooked food and her mother had agreed, delivering to her daughter every school lunch, hamburgers, fries and soft drink from a well-known fast food franchise. That situation was bad enough but it actually got worse.

This sweet girl was also allowed to choose her breakfast which usually consisted of white toast with jam or a chocolate spread. However if running late for school, then mum would pass through the drive-through of a fast food franchise for pancakes and syrup on the way. This child was eating all 'dead' food, full of sugar and chemicals and her young body was literally starving for healthy nutrients, enzymes, vitamins, minerals and fibre.

So we discussed the importance of fresh fruit and vegetables – 'living food' – while I did Bowen on my young client. Her sessions were designed to help with her constipation, relieve stress, take the pressure off her knees and lower back to relieve her pain. We talked about how soft drink and flavoured milk are not the same as water as they are often high in sugar and chemicals which do not help with pain, stress and anxiety. The importance of movement and exercise for a healthy body was also discussed.

Because of my personal experience with pain and as a therapist, I am highly body aware. I've noticed I get body aches if I've been overworking or not looking after myself properly. Usually I have great stamina but that can start to wane if I'm not eating fresh 'live' food, exercising, meditating or having some regular Bowen to keep my body working effectively. It's a better idea to focus on prevention and deal with issues early rather than letting them develop and become entrenched. Part of resolving pain issues quickly is improving the quality of your food and water.

Quality Water

There's no denying that we are dealing with more chemicals every day in our air, food and water. While chemicals in treated town water have generally made it safe to drink there are concerns about what this constant exposure to such a mix of chemicals is doing to our bodies.

My personal experience is that I feel more energised, mentally clearer and physically better when I drink filtered water and I can definitely taste the difference. Once you have been regularly drinking filtered water you can taste the chemicals when you drink tap water, even in coffee and tea. The chemicals in treated water may also contribute to an acid-type environment in the body which can aggravate pain levels.

Several years ago, I was treating a council worker who was employed at the local government water treatment plant. I was talking to him about the importance of hydration and he just laughed. He told me he had a science degree and knew exactly what was in our town water and as a consequence he only drank tank, rainwater or natural spring water.

He talked about the quality of the water before it's treated, what is floating around in it and the pollutants, toxins and pesticides that feed into the river from nearby businesses, mining industry and farms. He told me about the volume of chemicals needed to make the water reasonably safe and how at the end of the working week, on Friday afternoons they would dump extra chemicals into the water supply to last over the weekend. So he advised that tap water was particularly potent and strong with chemicals on a Saturday morning.

Coincidentally the weekend before I met and treated this client, my husband and I had cleaned out our large fish tank which contained big, beautiful goldfish (several years old). It was Saturday morning and within a couple of hours of putting our healthy fish into the cleaned tank, they were all floating upside down, dead. We were devastated.

At the time, we couldn't work out what had gone wrong except that we usually cleaned the tank on a Sunday afternoon. My client told me never to clean fish tanks, fill up water bottles, etc. on a Saturday morning precisely for that reason. After treating him and hearing what he had to say, my family always uses water filters or spring water as much as possible.

Keep Hydrated!

A body in pain is usually highly acidic and this can increase from dehydration, consuming 'dead' and overprocessed foods and from chronic stress, etc. If we can start to bring the body towards a more natural state by drinking quality water, eating fresh food and green vegetables, handling our stress levels, etc., that can have an amazing impact on pain levels. This is something simple that you can do to help yourself.

Be mindful of your environment. Some of us live in a warm tropical climate where the heat and humidity encourages voluminous sweating and if you are working outside in the heat you will lose even more. Replacing your fluids and electrolytes is important. Dehydration can make you tired, more prone to accidents, cramping and increasing pain levels. Dehydration has also been implicated in arthritis, joint pain, angina, diabetes, asthma, high blood pressure, headaches, stress, depression, gastric pain and constipation.

In summer, I see more clients in clinic complaining about cramping. Usually in the extremities such as the feet and legs and while physical release of those tight and contracted muscles through Bowen and massage deal with the immediate pain and distress, ensuring your water intake is adequate is also important for prevention and ongoing management.

Of course the sweat you lose is not just water but also valuable minerals and electrolytes. I'm not a fan of soft drinks or sports drinks because generally they can be high in sugar and chemicals. You can make your own by adding fruit slices to water and a squeeze of fresh juice from orange, lemon or limes. If you are cramping, a pinch of Himalayan rock salt or a good sea or mineral salt may also be helpful to add. I love citrus fruits in my water and also alternate with a dose of Young Living's Ningxia Red which contains natural food sourced vitamins and minerals to help support a healthy lifestyle.

If you live in a cooler climate, you can still be dehydrated through exposure to cold dry air. Your skin dries out and even your lungs can release moisture as you breathe. So whether you are becoming dehydrated from the heat or the cold, your body will automatically redirect fluids to your essential organs which is a survival mechanism. However this can impact on your extremities so that if you have poor circulation (or lymphatic issues) in your hands, feet, arms and legs, your pain levels can be amplified. Drinking water is important – no matter where you live!

Just to clarify, when talking about quality water for hydration and pain relief, I'm not talking about coffee, soft drink or soda, cordial, milk drinks or liquid foods because that is how your body processes those things – as foods. As soon as you add sugar, milk or chemicals to your water, your body no longer sees it as just water. Your water intake is in addition to those liquid foods.

Strong coffee, caffeinated soft drinks and alcohol can also dehydrate so you will need additional water if you consume those things. Do you drink diet drinks or beverages with artificial sweetener? Many people go to the toilet more often if they have been drinking them in quantity. It's the body's desperate attempt to flush toxins out but in the process it can also release calcium and minerals from bones and joints which can aggravate pain.

Some clients justify why they don't drink water by joking, "Fish pee in water so why would I drink it?" And while it may be a joke, that person is usually chronically dehydrated and experiencing high pain levels. Yes that's hilarious!

Artificial Sweeteners

As mentioned in Chapter One when battling my MS diagnosis, I noticed that my joints were 'clicky' and noisy (in addition to the excruciating pain). In my high school years, diet soft drink was introduced into the Australian market and so basically since I was 16 I'd had a regular intake of diet soft drink each week day. The dangers of diet soft drinks were still too new for me to find any research at that time (this was before the internet) but I instinctively stopped drinking them when I decided to eat fresh and clean.

I noticed that the noise and some pain in my joints disappeared within a couple of weeks of eliminating diet soft drinks. Even to this day, if I very occasionally have a diet soft drink (maybe once or twice a year as part of me wants to test if I still react the same way), the 'clicking' is back the next day and it lasts for several days. *Joint Health* magazine in the article 'How Can Soft Drinks Worsen Your Osteoarthritis and Joint Pain?' agrees:

> *Despite what most soda manufacturers want you to believe, those diet versions of their drinks are just as hazardous to your health ... drinking soda on a regular basis can have a serious impact on your body's ability to maintain good joint health. Those suffering from osteoarthritis and joint pain need to take the time to cut these drinks out of their day. The results will be decreased joint pain, better prevention of the development of their arthritis, and much more. Switching to a healthy drink will have numerous other health impacts as well including things like better heart health, reduced cancer risk, and weight loss. But it will also help you manage your pain within your joints.*

From research now available, artificial sweeteners have been implicated in many nerve and health conditions and may leach nutrients from the body having a detrimental effect on the joints, bones and kidneys. Dr Oz warns of the dangers of artificial sweeteners and advises that the common ones such as aspartame (in most diet soft drinks), sucralose (often extended with unidentified fillers) and saccharin (made from petroleum) are being shunned now by a more informed public. However the soft drink industry in response has invented new names for its problem sweeteners to make it more difficult for consumers to identify, so watch out for Equal, NutraSweet, Sweet N Low, Splenda, Natrulose, Smart Sweet, Isomaltitol, Sugar Alcohol and Maltitol Syrup as well as others.

Just a quick word about another liquid toxin – alcohol. It contains empty calories devoid of any good nutrition but also can deplete valuable minerals and nutrients, causing dehydration. It burdens the liver and kidneys and also from a pain point of view increases your chances of accidents and re-injury.

But wait there's more! Alcohol also makes your body more acidic and while under its influence you may be temporarily less aware of your pain, when you sober up you will experience it in full force. If you are serious about long term pain relief, daily or excessive consumption has to go.

If you are currently addicted to your soft drink, artificial sweeteners or alcohol, you can start to wean yourself by:

- increasing your 'quality' water consumption. Have a glass of water before or after every alcoholic or soft drink.

- increase support to your liver and kidneys. Raw foods such as green vegetables and salads are kinder to your liver and raw beetroot, grated in salads or juiced, is traditionally thought to support the kidneys. Drinking good water also helps the functioning of these important organs.

- gradually decreasing your consumption of these pain aggravators.

- replace with healthy options such as herbal teas, naturally flavoured water with fresh fruit, kombucha or fresh vegetable juices etc

Herbal Teas

A healthier drink alternative you might like to try are herbal teas which can be consumed hot or cold. I personally love Young Living's Slique Tea which contains exotic ingredients such as Oolong Jade Tea, Ocotea and Frankincense powder.

Also just released, is a special herbal tea range I've formulated to support people on their wellness journey. If you'd like to know more, please visit: www.DrugFreePainReliefBook.com.

Vitamin C

In Chapter One, I mentioned my use of high quality vitamin C supplements. Back then, I had to place a special order with my chemist to get calcium or sodium ascorbate powder with bioflavonoids including hesperidin and rutin. In those days it was very expensive but I was investing in my health, my life and so I was just thankful to be able to get it.

I took multiple doses throughout the day and it worked well for me. I'm not a big fan of tablets generally as you don't know what fillers or binders they contain. I personally prefer capsules or powders that can be put into a healthy smoothie, fresh vegetable or fruit juice.

Sometimes vitamins can be really cheap but that's often when they have been made from artificial or synthetic ingredients. Ideally anything we ingest should be as close to natural food as possible. If you have pain and a stressed body, it doesn't need the extra load of processing unnatural chemicals.

Because I get naturally occurring vitamin C from the fresh food I eat and my daily dose of Young Living's Ningxia Red, I don't necessarily take a supplement every day now, but I will take it at certain times of the year. For example, before I go travelling and then after, if I've been exposed to people really unwell or if I'm feeling stressed or rundown.

When I was 23 I caught Ross River Fever (polyarthritis) from a mosquito bite and at that time there was no treatment or cure. My doctor advised rest, painkillers and to be prepared to be unable to work for a couple of months. He advised that when it eventually passed, it would regularly come back if I were to get tired and run down. It was déjà vu – my joints were so sore and stiff and as with my MS diagnosis, I had to crawl up and down stairs on my hands and knees. But again I was determined to beat it.

Lady Cilento to the rescue. She wrote about Ross River Fever in her book *The Cilento Way* and how mega-doses of vitamin C had the potential to help with that and other conditions such as glandular fever, arthritis, shingles and infective hepatitis. So I went back to taking large daily doses of vitamin C (with hesperidin and rutin) and it worked brilliantly!

Within a few days of taking it, my joint aches and pains had started to dissipate and by two weeks I could walk up and down our stairs and had started back at work. I kept taking the vitamin C powder for several months to make sure I had cleared the virus from my system and I have never had a relapse.

About six months later our family pet, a dachshund dog named Skippy was walking very painfully and was struggling to move her short legs. She would normally run up our back stairs to sit at our kitchen door but was no longer able to do so. We took her to the vet who said Skippy had dog arthritis and there was nothing he could do to help. I decided to try my vitamin C powder with her and sprinkled it on her dinner every day. Within two weeks she was back to her old self and walking up and down our back stairs easily.

Vitamin C also has the potential to help with other pain conditions. In *Good Health in the 21st Century*, Dr Carole Hungerford advises that it helps with the repair of collagen and therefore can assist with damaged knees and ankles as well as associated conditions such as fatigue and depression.

Vitamin D

Vitamin D is one of those vitamins that you generally can get naturally through exposure to sunlight. Depending on where you live, your lifestyle and your physical condition you might also need to supplement.

There are many variables. You could work or spend your day mostly indoors and rarely see the sun. Your geographical location and the time and season of the year can also dictate how much natural vitamin D you get exposed to.

Generally during winter people get less vitamin D due to shorter daylight hours and wearing more clothing and this situation can increase pain levels. Alternatively, have you noticed how people feel so much happier and are more active in the summer months?

Vitamin D helps support strong healthy bones and a low level can contribute to muscle, joint and bone aches. If you have low vitamin D you may find that you are using more pain medication or that it becomes less effective. To offset that situation, consider getting outside at least three times a week and utilising natural and free sunlight. It's a simple and easy thing to do to support yourself in having a pain free life.

As a side note, Dr Michael Holick in *The Vitamin D Solution*, writes about how low levels have been implicated in back and joint pain as well as autoimmune conditions such as MS, type 1 diabetes and rheumatoid arthritis. Living in areas closer to the equator or getting outside to get more frequent sun exposure and eating foods rich in vitamin D can decrease your chances of such conditions.

Of course if you can't regularly get out in natural sunlight, there are vitamin D supplements available. I personally use Young Living's OmegaGize that contains natural vitamin D, wild harvested Omega-3 fish oil and CoQ10 – so convenient to have just the one supplement that covers all those things. If you have any questions or would like to access Young Living products, please contact the person who introduced you to Young Living, their details are listed in Recommended Resources at the back of this book. If you haven't been introduced by anyone, visit: *www.yldist.com/suzannemctierbrowne*.

Magnesium

A generally safe non-toxic mineral that can ease muscle tightness and tension, cramping and allow a good night's sleep. Often people in pain get constipated. That can happen from taking pain medications or from the continual stress and so magnesium will normally help to deal with that complaint also.

Magnesium has many important body functions which include nerve transmission, calcium and potassium uptake, bone formation and regulating the acid–alkaline balance in the body. Deficiencies in this important mineral can impact on your health beyond chronically tight muscles and can contribute to coronary heart disease, obesity, fatigue and impaired brain function. It is worth noting that chocolate cravings can be an indication of magnesium deficiency.

It is excreted by the body if you are ingesting too much so that makes it a safe mineral supplement to have at home. Dr Sandra Cabot in *Magnesium – The Miracle Mineral* lists a whole range of other pain-impacting conditions that magnesium can assist such as adrenal gland exhaustion, anxiety, arthritis, constipation, depression, fibromyalgia, irritability, migraines, MS, muscle cramps/weakness and stress. It's something I've been taking regularly for the past decade and many of my clients have also found useful in supporting their recovery from pain.

Magnesium can be applied topically in gels or creams, or can be taken in supplement form. The better utilised and absorbed forms in supplements tend to be magnesium orotate, magnesium amino acid chelate and magnesium aspartate. Powders that combine different types of magnesium with Taurine can also be useful.

White Sugar

Have you heard the term 'the white death'? It generally refers to the consumption of white, processed sugar (and white refined flour) which are devoid of minerals and nutrients and can be a pain aggravator. There's been a lot written about the high levels of sugar in our modern day diet and how it can contribute to conditions such as diabetes, weight issues, cancer etc.

In *Outsmart Sugar*, Tara Mitchell writes, "One Coke raises the blood sugar to five times normal level, for at least four hours."

Consuming refined sugars can also feed any virus, bacteria or moulds in the body so if you have yeast infections, colds, flu, candida, etc., you might like to consider greatly reducing your sugar intake. I've also found personally and in clinic that it can increase pain levels. In *Take Control of Your Health and Escape the Sickness Industry*, Elaine Hollingsworth agrees:

Sugar leaches the body of precious minerals and vitamins because of the heavy demands its detoxification and elimination make on the entire system. It produces an over-acid condition, and more and more minerals are required from the body in the attempt to rectify the imbalance. To protect the blood, so much calcium is leached from the teeth and bones that osteoporosis and decay, and weakening of the entire body, results ... Every ounce of sugar eaten reduces the ability of the body to resist infection, because it damages the immune system, leaving the body prey to every possible illness, including arthritis, heart disease, arteriosclerosis, atherosclerosis and cancer.

Men with osteoarthritis of the knee may find it beneficial to avoid sugar rich soft drinks. Researcher and Assistant Professor of Medicine at Harvard Medical School and Associate Biostatistician at Brigham and Women's Hospital in Boston, Dr Bing Lu, conducted a study on knee osteoarthritis with more than 2,000 people and found that men had greater risk of worsening their condition the more they regularly drank soft drinks or soda:

Soft drinks worsen knee osteoarthritis independently of the wear and tear on the joints caused by carrying around excess weight ... After taking into account BMI and other risk factors for knee osteoarthritis, men who drank five or more soft drinks a week had twice as much narrowing of joint space compared with men who did not drink sugary soda.

Now I am not perfect and I have to admit that I do battle a chocolate addiction, particularly if under prolonged stress. But I can also go for long periods of time without sugar and feel so good when I do. I have been pain free now for decades because I reduce sugar as much as possible plus doing the other strategies I list in this book.

Helpful Herbs

Introducing some fresh herbs into your daily diet may also help with reducing your pain. You can go to your local markets and buy fresh and locally grown, or grow your own. You can then control what pesticides and chemicals you are exposing your body.

I love making breakfast in the morning and walking out onto my patio to get a selection of homegrown basil, parsley, oregano, garlic chives and mint. Even smelling fresh herbs can help you feel good!

Following are some spices and herbs that are gaining popularity with pain relief:

> *Warning/disclaimer: The following culinary herbs are used in cooking and of course millions of people have eaten these herbs for thousands of years with no ill effects. However, if you have a medical condition and take prescription medications, you should check with your doctor or pharmacist. For example, turmeric and ginger may thin the blood.*

Turmeric – the Queen of Spices

If you like curry, turmeric (curcuma longa) is the spice that gives it strong golden colour and unique flavour. Research indicates that turmeric has natural anti-inflammatory qualities and may assist with circulation. Turmeric has been used traditionally in Indian and Chinese medicine for muscle pain and joint inflammation, etc. Dr Joseph Mercola advises it's active ingredient – curcumin, has been found to inhibit and reduce the two enzymes in the body that can cause inflammation – cyclooxygenase-2 (COX2) and 5-lipoxygenase (5-LOX), as well as other enzymes that have been implicated:

A 2006 study also found that a turmeric extract composed of curcuminoids (curcumin is the most investigated curcuminoid) blocked inflammatory pathways, effectively preventing the launch of a protein that triggers swelling and pain.

I use this spice daily. I sprinkle it on my eggs in the morning for breakfast and use it in my other meals such as salad, casseroles and soups. For better uptake and absorption, it's good to combine turmeric with black pepper. It's so easy just to have a little each day.

Make your own special seasoning with a selection of organic turmeric, curry powder, Himalayan salt, ground pepper and dried herbs – wonderful for sprinkling over cooked vegetables or meat. Just be careful, turmeric has lovely colour which can easily transfer onto your clothes or white surfaces.

Of course there are other ways you can take turmeric – in supplements or in 'golden milk', an ancient Ayurvedic drink. There are numerous golden milk recipes around using variations of turmeric, black pepper, coconut oil, ginger, cinnamon, honey etc. You can make up your own golden paste which you keep in the fridge and then just use a little each time to make your golden milk.

You can also use raw turmeric and ginger (some think it's more effective). Of course you should do your own research and find the best recipe for you but for your information, here's a simple recipe I use:

Golden Paste

1/4 cup organic turmeric powder

1/2 cup of filtered water

1 teaspoon black pepper

3 tablespoons virgin coconut oil (cold pressed).

Preferably in a small stainless steel pot, cook the turmeric, water and black pepper until it forms a smooth paste on medium heat, stirring so it doesn't burn. Remove from heat, cool slightly and thoroughly mix in the coconut oil. Store the golden paste in a small glass jar in the refrigerator for up to two weeks (if it develops a metallic taste, it's been stored too long so throw it out).

Use your golden paste to make your golden milk drink or you can take a half a teaspoon mixed with a little honey to taste. For severe pain, you could try two serves a day. Golden milk is becoming popular to have before going to bed and is thought to also help with a good night's sleep.

Golden Milk

1/4 – 1/2 teaspoon of Golden Paste

1 cup milk (can be coconut, almond or cow, preferably not homogenised)

Ginger, vanilla and/or cinnamon to taste (optional)

Honey (or natural sweetener) to taste (optional)

Preferably in a stainless steel pot, gently mix and heat to steaming (but do not boil) 1 cup of milk with up to 1/2 teaspoon of golden paste. Remove from heat and add optional vanilla, ginger, cinnamon and/or honey to taste.

Ginger

Ginger, another natural anti-inflammatory, has been used to help with muscle pain for thousands of years in Chinese medicine. Ginger has other uses and may assist with stomach conditions, nausea, arthritis and headaches etc. *Healthy and Natural World* reports:

> *Ginger contains powerful anti-inflammatory substances called gingerols. These have been tested in various research of rheumatic diseases such as osteoarthritis or rheumatoid arthritis where the participants reported a gradual reduction of pain, improving agility and movement and reduction in swelling when using ginger regularly.*

A spice easy to incorporate into your regular food such as marinades, sweets, desserts and herbal tea. You can easily make your own ginger tea, grating some fresh ginger into your hot water, strain (if you want) and then sip. Ginger can also be applied topically in a compress, or ointment for stiff joints, pain and inflammation.

Valerian

An interesting herb with a long history, Valerian has been used by the Anglo-Saxons since the Middle Ages and was popular in Britain for neuralgic pain, insomnia, hysteria etc. In both world wars, it was commonly used for traumatised soldiers and civilians. Dr Oz advises:

> *Called nature's tranquiliser, valerian has been used for centuries to regulate the nervous system and relieve insomnia, tension, irritability, stress, and anxiety. Valerian is also a natural pain reliever that reduces sensitivity of the nerves.*

Valerian can also be helpful to get a good night's rest which is so important when you are battling pain.

Young Living Essential Oils

Some people are very disciplined and prepare fresh organic or local food each day – and if that is you, well done! Healthy eating is very important to help reduce pain. Nutrition supplements can be an additional easy and practical way to support your health.

After years of researching and trying many, I prefer high quality plant or food based whenever possible (not synthetic or artificial) and therefore choose to use Young Living products. I've visited several Young Living farming operations in Ecuador, USA (Utah and Idaho) and Darwin, Australia, and have seen personally the amount of expertise and quality control that goes into making their therapeutic grade essential oils and supplements.

My favourite energy drink is Ningxia Red – how my life has changed from having it daily. I had been working in my clinic for several years and the demand was huge. Exhausted I finally decided that I needed to close clinic for a few weeks to recuperate. I had recently got my wholesale account with Young Living and was already using some of the essential oils but hadn't at that point tried Ningxia Red or the supplements. After a week of using them I quickly noticed a difference.

Because of my increased energy and stamina, I never closed clinic but kept on working. The improvement in mental clarity helped me make changes that allowed me to not overwork myself. It is amazing what can happen when you feed your body superior nutrition. Refer to Chapter Ten if you'd like more information. If you have any questions or would like to access Young Living products, please contact the person who introduced you (their details are listed in Recommended Resources at the back of this book). If no one introduced you, please visit: *www.yldist.com/suzannemctierbrowne*

I had a constant headache and neck tension for five weeks. Confusion was evident and this was the reason I came to consult Suzanne. In general I did not feel well. I have had three treatments with Suzanne and I feel so much alive and my mixed feelings and confusion have completely gone. My vision is so much clearer and I feel so well, noticed by the doctor and my family. Thank you Sue.   Janette V.

(NB: Janette had Bowen Therapy for structural correction and to release tight muscles. She also began taking Young Living supplements to support her health.)

But finally, don't take my word – do your own investigations. Ask questions, read books or research articles, try things and see how they work for you. Be your own body detective, be courageous and take action.

Here's the Truth:

That old saying "you can lead a horse to water but you can't make it drink" is true. Food and supplement choices are mentioned in this book and maybe your doctor or therapist has already spoken to you about these things, but you actually have to do it. YOU have to make a decision, take action and make the change. Just thinking about it doesn't cut it!

The first priority is to eat raw and living food to help provide your body with the natural energy and vitality to heal and restore healthy tissue and function. Eating high quality fresh food and staying hydrated with quality water is so important achieving and maintaining a pain free life.

Cooked and over-processed food is literally 'dead' food and has little nutrient or 'live' energy value for your body particularly if you are unwell or dealing with chronic pain. Don't eat rubbish and then expect a quality outcome.

> *"Your body is your responsibility – your food and lifestyle choices help create the body you deserve."*
>
> **Suzanne McTier-Browne**

Final Word:

I've yet to meet anyone who does everything perfectly. If you do decide to indulge occasionally, please do so with no guilt! Just relax and enjoy it – don't stress! Make the decision to eat better tomorrow and try to make the majority of your food choices healthy!

Beware the Toxic Environment

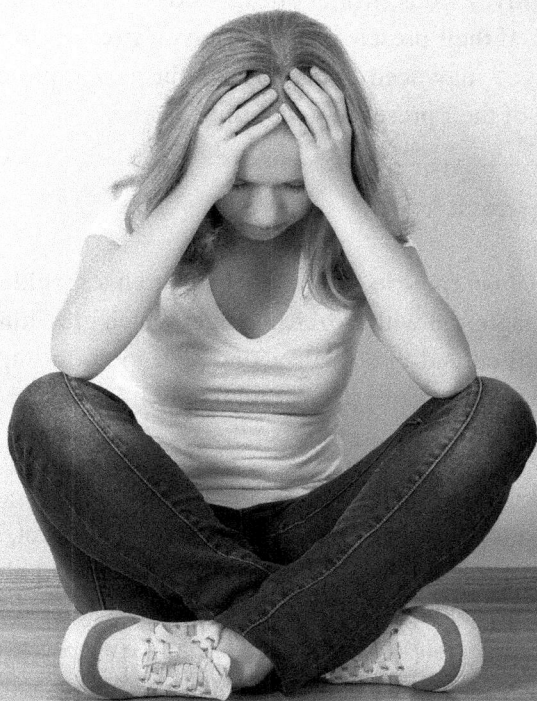

CHAPTER 7

Beware the Toxic Environment

> *"Beware the 4 Ps of the toxic environment – People and Pollution (Places and Personal) which can increase your pain both physically and psychologically."*
>
> **Suzanne McTier-Browne**

Let's look at the first and most difficult to manage – people. Are there toxic people in your environment? Interactions with such people can definitely affect your physical and emotional pain. Toxic people in your life could be family, friends, work colleagues or someone you come into frequent contact. If their presence is causing you stress or to sabotage or self-harm, then you may need to take back your power, protect yourself and take control of their presence in your life.

Case Study – Toxic Wife!

A quiet, gentle man came to see me. He had hurt his shoulder about a year earlier, diagnosed with frozen shoulder which gave him intense pain. He was tired and in despair about what to do to improve his condition. He had tried everything and finally his friend (a client of mine) had told him to see me.

A physical assessment found structural imbalances, contracted muscles plus a highly restricted neck range of movement, he could barely turn his head. After the first session, he regained almost full range of movement in his neck, his posture greatly improved and he said the pain in his shoulder had reduced 50%. That was a great result for someone not physically fit and who had a chronic condition.

His second visit the next week got his shoulder moving, his range improved to 45 degrees. He was delighted and came back for a third session where he improved even further and could move his arm to 90 degrees. By this stage the pain he had experienced for the past year was mostly gone. His skin pallor had improved, he was standing taller, had more energy and he was smiling – a lot. He excitedly rebooked.

When he returned for his fourth session, he brought his wife. As soon as I saw them walk through the door, you could see this was not a happy couple dynamic. The smiling excited man from last week was gone, his posture was stooped and he followed meekly behind his wife. She however was excited. "I just had to come and say thanks. Now his shoulder is working I have a big list of things he can do at home. You know, he hasn't done anything for the past year!"

During his session she continually talked loudly at him and to me. He responded well and came off the table with almost full range of movement in his shoulder – that made his wife even more excited. I strongly cautioned about the need for him to be gentle with his shoulder, not do anything too physical and no heavy lifting as he had no movement at all for the previous year and it takes time to rebuild muscle tone etc. They booked a follow-up appointment .

It was so sad to see him walk in that next week. His wife did not come and you could see he wanted to vent. He had reinjured his shoulder working through the chores on her list and he was angry – at her. His shoulder now could only move half the range it did the previous week.

Apparently he'd been nagged (his words) into clearing their backyard, cutting down trees and digging up the stumps. All that with a shoulder that hadn't even moved in the year prior to treatment. I was horrified – this was the exact opposite of what I had advised. However it was clear to see the toxic dynamics in their relationship had instigated the re-injury of his shoulder. She may have been loud, dominant or even a bully in their relationship but he did not seem to stand up for himself. He chose to not speak up and protect his shoulder.

He deliberately got stuck into that list of chores, against advice, to teach his wife a lesson (passive aggressively). He could have protected himself and perhaps said "the chores will have to wait" or "we'll pay someone to do them". However he decided (perhaps subconsciously) to injure himself so that he had an excuse and would not physically be able to continue to do the things she was telling him. It seems he wasn't prepared to face her and say NO. Of course ultimately his body is his choice and if someone chooses re-injury there is nothing anyone else can do.

If someone is impacting on your pain or physical or emotional health, it is up to you to take some kind of positive action and start to control the situation. Some basic strategies you might like to try if you are dealing with toxic people are:

✓ Draw a line in the sand! Stand up for yourself and communicate your needs clearly. Have you actually talked to them and let them know what you want and need? They can't change how they deal with you unless you let them know how it makes you feel. Maybe they don't realise how their behaviour affects you – you have to articulate your feelings.

✓ If they don't care about what you say and won't change their behaviour, you can change how you deal with them! Be honest with yourself and your pain. If someone is having a detrimental effect on you, you may need to restrict the amount or type of contact with them. In severe cases, you may need to remove contact temporarily or even permanently. If you don't prioritise your pain relief and health, why should anyone else?

✓ If you can't disconnect from them totally then perhaps you can manage and contain. Put boundaries around your interactions with them and control the contact:

- Don't see them alone.

- Meet in a protected environment or in the company of other people which can diffuse the effect on you – they may also behave better in front of other people.

- Perhaps don't communicate face to face if it causes you distress. You could do so by text, email, phone messages or through other people.

- Only interact when your strength and energy is high.

- Keep interactions short and schedule at a time that suits you. Being in control will help you deal with the situation more positively.

You can also support and increase your own positive energy by:

- consuming fresh 'live' food

- drinking quality water

- have structural correction bodywork

- taking quality supplements

- regular meditation

- daily stretching and exercise

- deep breathing

- positive thinking and affirmations

- being out in nature

- being around happy people and positive, fun environments.

Negative people in your life can be very toxic. Sometimes these 'energy vampires' who drain you may not know that they are having that effect. They may not be intentionally draining you and in that case honesty maybe your best policy. Consider telling them the situation and that you can't see them until you are stronger or they change and become more positive and supportive.

However sometimes there are 'energy vampires' in your life who are well aware of the effect they have on you and 'attack' you intentionally. If you really have to be around that type of person then you should take steps to protect yourself. Some strategies you might like to try before you come into contact:

• Remember you are powerful. Set protective intentions for your day and before you see those toxic people. This could be as simple as sitting quietly, closing your eyes, taking deep breaths and visualising what you want to happen. See yourself as strong, energised and protected. Access the warrior within you!

• You could visualise surrounding yourself with a powerful barrier that insulates you from negative words and energies. Some people visualise a golden translucent egg that cocoons and protects, keeping out negative energies. Some imagine a comforting cloak that swirls around your shoulders and provides protection. Some visualise hugging a beautiful strong tree that is keeping you safe and grounded. Just use whatever mental imagery that makes you feel safe and comfortable.

• If I'm going to be around negative people or in situations that make me feel uncomfortable, I like to use some high frequency essential oils. Some of my favourites are Young Living's White Angelica, Joy, Valor, Frankincense or Sacred Mountain. I might inhale them or wear them as a perfume to feel strong and confident. Holding the bottle 5–10 cm above your head and let a drop fall onto your crown, falling through the energetic chakra layers can also be a beautiful way to balance and strengthen.

- You can even place good intentions and positive affirmations into your favourite essential oil. Then when you wear it and inhale the scent, you are easily reminded of your positive intent.

- Diffusing essential oils in your room can also raise the frequencies and energies in your space and make you feel more positive and peaceful.

- Perhaps buy yourself a quartz crystal or whatever type of gem stone that resonates with you (makes you feel good) and then carry it around with you. Keep it in your pocket, handbag or even wear inside your clothes so you can touch it, be comforted and supported when you need it.

If you have been caught off-guard, there are some things you might like to try to shake off that negative energy:

- Go for a swim, water is a great cleanser.

- Go for a walk or run out in nature, get some fresh air in your lungs and wind on your face.

- Sit outside in the sunshine (or the rain) and let the healing power of nature restore you.

- Exercise, going to the gym, playing sport or any focused activity can be beneficial.

- Have a shower, wash your hair and visualise all that negativity just washing away down the drain.

- Imagine or visualise a beautiful 'positive energy' waterfall washing down and cleansing you.

- Inhale or wear your favourite essential oil.

- Earth or ground yourself by walking in bare feet on the grass or sand. You could even lie down on the grass and just relax.

Often when you stay strong and positive, toxic people will feel uncomfortable around your good energy and they will leave your space or even stay but begin to change for the better. Either way that's a great outcome!

When you are dealing with negative or toxic people it can be a bit of a mind game. Set boundaries, protect and stand up for yourself, be strong. Generally no one can hurt you unless you let them!

Now to clarify, I'm not talking about physically abusive people. No one has the right to physically hurt or abuse you. I do not take such situations lightly and you should not either. If your situation is so toxic that it involves physical abuse then you need immediate professional assistance (this also applies to severe psychological abuse). Your doctor or the police may be your first step and you need to be very honest about your situation. People can only help if you ask or seek help. Some useful contacts are included at the back of this book in Recommended Resources.

So if being around toxic people can have negative effect on your pain and health, then the reverse is also true. Being around positive, happy people can help ease your pain, loneliness and anxiety. Be mindful about who you keep in your company. Are your friends positive and cheerful? Notice the language they use when talking to you and about you. Do they support and encourage you?

Bruce Lipton in his book, *The Biology of Belief* details research that has shown that people in a healthy positive relationship and having physical contact with that loved one can lower blood pressure, alleviate stress, improve health and decrease physical pain. Loving family and friends are very important in supporting your pain relief journey.

The Second P – Pollution (Places and Personal)!

Pollution and toxic chemicals in the environment (and in us) is such a huge issue that it has had numerous research and books devoted to it. *Slow Death by Rubber Duck* written by Rick Smith and Bruce Lourie, gives a summary of the problem:

> *Back in 1991, a gathering of international experts first
> warned us about chemicals that have the potential to disrupt
> the hormone systems of animals and humans ... Hormone
> disruptions, like climate change, is a spin-off from society's
> addiction to fossil fuels. The damaging effects of hormone-
> disrupting chemicals on fertility, the brain and behaviour quite
> possibly make them a more imminent threat to humankind ...
> We are now into the fourth generation of people exposed to
> toxic chemicals from before conception through to adulthood,
> and statistics tell us that humankind is under siege.*

Though extremely important, the immensity of this subject cannot
adequately be dealt with in this chapter (or book). Also if you are in pain,
you probably don't have the energy to read in detail about this subject,
therefore here is some practical information which is within your power
to deal.

Your home and workplace are the two places you spend most of your
time and will tend to be the two main areas where you would be regularly
exposed to toxins. Some of those toxins will be obvious, such smoke,
rising damp and mould. Some will be less obvious such as pesticides,
asbestos, lead and toxic building materials.

Some pollution is electromagnetic energy based and can come through
exposure to technology such as mobile phones, computers, power
lines and some medical equipment. There is still debate as to what are
safe levels of exposure and the possible effect on the human body of
accumulated contact but any 'toxin' may increase stress, decrease energy,
impair normal function and increase pain levels. Living in a clean and
toxin free environment as much as possible can help channel your body's
energies into healing and becoming pain free.

Mobile phones, used frequently by most people, emit radiofrequency
(RF) radiation which in May 2011 was classified by the World Health
Organization (WHO) as "possibly carcinogenic for humans, based on an

increased risk for glioma, a type of brain cancer". If you would like to reduce potential exposure to RF, here are some simple things to consider:

- Maintain some distance or use a physical barrier or container like a handbag or briefcase to carry your phone rather than place it directly on your body. Read your phone specifications, it will usually state the safe distance away from the body it should be operated (varies depending on the model). If you want to keep your phone in your pocket, you have options like putting it in airplane or flight mode, or to turn it off when not in use.

- At night, if you sleep with your phone near your head, clasped in your hand or under your pillow, think about placing it away from the bed. It's also easy to turn off WiFi, bluetooth and data download options if you still want to use it as your alarm.

- Use the loud speaker function, head or earphones so you don't have to hold it close against your head. You can also try using maximum volume and holding it a safe distance away from your ear.

- The best reception for your phone is when you have the maximum number of bars so try to use it then. Anything that blocks reception and gives poor signal strength makes your phone work harder, use more power and emit more RF.

- Did you know most mobile phones are designed to let out more radiation at the back of the unit and less through the front because it is designed to be closer to your face? So which way do you put your phone in your pocket? Is the back of the phone always facing away from your body to reduce exposure?

- Many people use their tablet or laptop in bed, resting on their body. The last laptop I purchased had radiation warnings on the box and in the instructions it said to use it at a safe distance of at least 20 cm from the body, so I use mine on a desk. We use technology so frequently that we tend to become blasé but when the manufacturers give warnings, it makes sense to take notice!

Cleaning and decluttering your environment can also help immensely. Clutter, rubbish, dirt and dust can also hide toxins, moulds and pests from view. Thoroughly clean and open up windows for fresh air to circulate. Allowing natural sunlight into a home or work environment can also help.

Air filtering plants can improve air quality as shown in the 1989 NASA Clean Air Study. Common indoor plants were shown to naturally remove toxins such as benzene, formaldehyde, trichloroethylene and ammonia as well as absorbing carbon dioxide and releasing oxygen (normal plant functions). Researchers suggested at least one plant per 100 square feet of office or home area. Most useful plants were the Peace Lily (Spathiphyllum), Chrysanthemum or Florist's Daisy (Chrysanthemum morifolium), Snake Plant or Mother-in-law's Tongue (Sansevieria trifasciata), Red-edged Dracaena (Dracaena marginata) and common English or European Ivy (Hedera helix).

Mass media can also be toxic. Watching too much negative or depressing television, violent or scary horror movies and games etc puts your body into stress mode. Your heart rate elevates, your body goes into 'fight or flight' mode and starts producing stress hormones such as cortisol. The exact opposite of what you want if you are aiming to lower pain levels. Your body heals when it is relaxed, happy and feeling safe.

So the alternative of watching happy, positive and 'feel good' programs can have real benefit. Norman Cousins is the famous example of using positive media such as comedy shows and movies to heal and deal with pain. Norman was a respected editor of the *Saturday Review* and was known as a global peacemaker. He received the UN Peace Medal, hundreds of other awards plus 50 honorary doctorate degrees.

In 1964, he was diagnosed with a degenerative disease (ankylosing spondylitis) which caused constant pain and his doctor diagnosed as fatal. He left the hospital, booked into a hotel and while taking high doses of vitamin C watched continuously humorous movies and comedy shows. He famously claimed when medication did not help him, that ten minutes of laughter would give him two hours of pain-free sleep. His condition improved and he later returned to full-time work. His story inspired scientific research and he later wrote a book *An Anatomy of An Illness* which was made into a movie.

Let's now quickly visit some basic quantum physics. Everything in this world is a form of energy. You, me, this book, everything is in various states of matter vibrating at different frequencies. As energy beings we tend to be more comfortable with people or places that resonate or vibrate at a similar frequency – it's just science!

Depending on how observant and body aware you are, sometimes you may go to a place and instantly feel comfortable and at home (this can also happen with people). It just means you are resonating at similar frequencies and things go smoothly and easily. Vibration and frequency can help explain how your gut instinct, heart or body automatically knows what is best for you.

However if you go somewhere or meet someone and you instantly feel bad or uncomfortable, then it might be a good idea for you to consider leaving! You're not vibrating on the same level and things may tend to be more difficult. No judgement, it simply may not be good for you at that time (or maybe never). That's just quantum physics!

Body Testing Tools

Pulse Test

Shortly after beating my MS diagnosis and cleaning up my eating habits, I realised after eliminating diet soft drink that when I did occasionally indulge, my pulse rate would substantially increase around ten minutes later, and then stay elevated for an hour or so. Besides the increased pulse rate, I would feel very lethargic and go to the toilet frequently.

There was a similar spike in pulse rate after eating cheap chocolate and I put it down to a mild sensitivity reaction or my body letting me know that particular food or drink was not doing me good. My pulse never spikes like that after eating fresh fruit or a salad!

While I have never read it, this phenomenon is apparently confirmed in Dr Arthur Coca's book, *The Pulse Test*. I am aware of my pulse now after I eat new foods or maybe indulge in things I really shouldn't. It's an easy and practical way to test and gauge whether a food or substance is helping or hindering.

I'm not saying it is the only way but being body aware and using the pulse test might also help you identify other toxins in your environment. It doesn't cost you anything to try for yourself and observe the results.

Breath Test

Another method using body intuition is the breath test. Our bodies are very smart and respond to stimuli in our environment without our conscious thought. One of the ways is through changes in breathing patterns.

You've probably experienced when you are under threat, how your breathing automatically changes to become more shallow and rises high into your chest. That is a typical stress response to a 'threat' your body perceives and it happens without any conscious thought. On the flip side, when you feel happy and safe your breathing will naturally deepen and become more diaphragmatic or 'belly breathing'. You can use this phenomenon, the inherent intelligence of your body to also help with decisions and choices.

When you have to make a choice, just take a couple of quiet seconds, tune into your body and think about the options separately, noticing your breathing pattern with each one. As a beginner, you might find it easier to put a hand on your chest and the other on your stomach and then notice which hand moves most. As you become more body aware, you will just be able to notice where your breathing is focused.

So if a choice or the subject matter you are thinking about causes you to breathe deeply – 'belly breathing' – this means that your body does not see it as a threat. If the subject or choice makes you shallow breath into your chest, your body is indicating there is something threatening or unsettling.

You need to stay neutral when doing this test and not consciously direct your breathing to get or indicate the outcome you want.

My personal experience has been that the option that gives the more relaxed 'belly breathing' has usually been the right choice. If your breathing goes into shallow, chest breathing, then there maybe something in that option that causes your body stress. Sometimes a negative response can be changed to positive with a small change. You still of course have the power to decide whether you use the results or not.

The pulse and breath tests are just simple techniques that I use to give myself more information and hopefully make better decisions. It's just a light-hearted way to use body intuition. At times, I also use other techniques such as the body sway and eye tests. But of course, you don't have to use all or any of them. These are just tools you might like to try and see how they work for you. For a free video demonstration of the body tests mentioned in this book, visit: *www.DrugFreePainReliefBook.com*.

Personal Pollution

The skin is the body's largest organ of absorption and the personal items we use every day can further expose us to toxic chemicals. Numerous things such as soap, laundry detergent, fabric softener, shampoo, conditioner, insect sprays, synthetic perfume, deodorant, toothpaste, makeup, aftershave and moisturiser – the list is endless. One of the many reasons I'm an avid user of Young Living products is that I can access toxin free alternatives that help reduce my family's exposure.

If you would like to reduce toxic chemicals in the home, in Chapter Ten I show what Young Living products I use daily. If you have any questions or would like to access Young Living products, please contact the person who introduced you to Young Living (their details are listed in Recommended Resources at the back of this book). If no one introduced you, please visit: *www.yldist.com/suzannemctierbrowne*.

Case Study – The Toxic Client!

The vast majority of clients respond well and provide a constant stream of new clients through word-of-mouth referrals and I am so grateful for them. However occasionally I get a client who refuses to acknowledge positive improvement, which is a real shame (for them). They are so negative in their outlook that they ignore the truth.

An elderly man in his 70s shuffled into my clinic using a walking stick, stooped over and obviously in extreme pain. He told me the pain was constant and had used the walking stick for three years. Pain medications were not working for him he said and he'd tried everything but nothing had worked. He was grumpy and abrupt but sometimes people in pain come in angry and frustrated, they usually leave happier!

After the session, he walked a lot easier and his posture was noticeably straighter. When he walked out into reception, he actually forgot his walking stick and left it behind so he had obviously had improvement. His wife waiting for him, noticed the positive change immediately, got very excited and commented about how quickly he had responded. He growled at her and his response "it would have happened anyway" was totally dismissive and incorrect. He then walked out the door (quite easily I might add), leaving his wife to pay and to recover his walking stick.

She apologised profusely and desperately wanted to book another appointment but I told her that I wasn't going to treat him unless he really wanted my help. She said that he had been grumpy and rude for a long time, not just with her but the whole family. She was hopeful that since he was now walking better and obviously not in as much pain that his personality and demeanour would improve. She started to cry and said she didn't know how long she could continue to stay with him if he didn't change. I comforted her and then suggested that they should see his doctor in case his aggression was being caused by a complication or new medical condition.

So please make sure that you're not the one who is toxic. Sometimes people in chronic pain can be angry and miserable. Are you are making life hard for everyone around you? Do people come to see you happy but then after spending time with you, leave depressed and miserable?

What kind of impact is your attitude having on your loved ones? Be honest, do you raise them up or pull them down? Just because you're battling pain at this time doesn't mean you have to bring down everyone around you.

It is also really important to be truthful and acknowledge positive improvement, no matter how small. It is a recognition that there can be positive change and is an important contribution to the healing process. Frequently people can get trapped in an all-consuming cycle of pain (refer to Chronic Pain Cycle Diagram, Chapter Two), depression and negative thought patterns. Focusing on your pain, can become habitual and then a reinforced behaviour.

It does take effort and commitment to turn around that "pain train" but where you put your attention grows bigger and stronger. You get to choose whether that is positive and puts you on the path to recovery and pain relief, or whether it's negative and continues to spiral you downwards into despair. Focusing on your recovery, being grateful for any improvements and being positive also makes you more comfortable to be around. As a bonus, being pleasant, you may attract even more support from family and friends.

And finally here's a **CRAP** (Chronic Really Awful Pain) poem!

Sometimes life is **CRAP**!

Can't **R**est, **A**nother **P**ain

Can **R**eally **A**nnoy **P**eople

Could **R**ile **A**ngry **P**eople

Rules are simple

Pain is a pimple

Crap in, crap out

Eat crap, become crap!

Hang around crappy people

You become the same – crappy!

Have crappy habits

You will stay in pain and be crappy!

But focus on your blessings

Be positive and you can

Celebrate **R**elief **A**nd **P**rogress!

(Ok, now you know I have a weird sense of humour and this is definitely not my finest writing but being able to laugh at myself helped keep me going during the tough times. If you feel offended by the above, maybe try writing your own CRAP poem and send it to me. I would love to read it!)

CHAPTER 8

Relax and Take a Big Breath

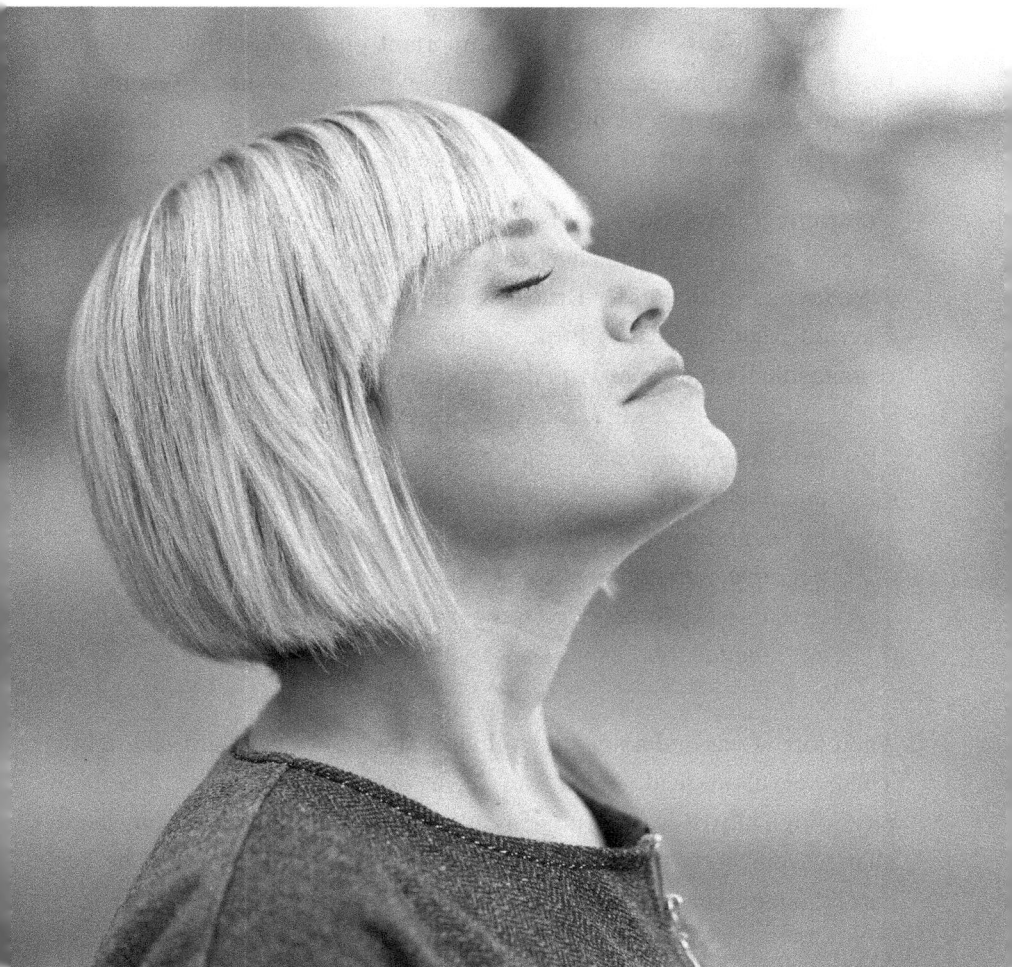

CHAPTER 8

Relax and Take a Big Breath!

> *"Mind matters! Your current pain is the result of past negative events plus your response and now daily thoughts and choices, both consciously and subconsciously."*
>
> **Suzanne McTier-Browne**

Previously discussed were some important physical and psychological factors that can increase pain so dealing with those issues if you haven't already done so may be in your best interest. But there is still one really important contributor that deserves more attention – mind matters!

Controlling stress and negative thought patterns can have a big impact on pain levels and if unchecked can aggravate existing conditions. In *The Biology of Belief*, Dr Bruce Lipton reports that Dr Herbert Benson, Harvard Medical School Professor of Medicine, found that stress was responsible for the majority of doctor visits (up to 90%). Dr Lipton writes:

> *Positive perceptions of the mind enhance health by engaging immune functions, while inhibition of immune activities by negative perceptions can precipitate disease. Those negative perceptions can also create debilitating, chronic psychological stress that has a profound and negative impact on gene function.*

Therefore stress and a negative mindset should not be dismissed lightly. These psychological states can have massive impact on the body physiologically. Research now shows that over time you can physically change your body with your thoughts. It really makes sense to be very careful about what you think.

When we 'change our beliefs', we change the blood's neurochemical composition, which then initiates a complementary change in the body's cells. The function of the mind is to create coherence between our beliefs and the reality we experience.

Memories, repeated rehearsal of trauma and the perception of the seriousness of the original injury can also prolong and exacerbate the pain experience. The more you think about it the worse it gets. It's a far better strategy to focus on the present and not dwell on the past.

Taking positive action and concentrating on recovery strategies can be both a welcome distraction and generate positive results. Research on chronic low back pain has also shown mind relaxation and calming techniques such as meditation and yoga to be effective pain strategies. Michael Woodhead writes in the article 'Meditation and Yoga Better For Low Back Pain Than Usual Care':

Meditation and yoga offer as much benefit for people with chronic low back pain as their usual care which could include NSAIDs (non-steroidal anti-inflammatory drugs, e.g. ibuprofen), a US trial suggests. Patients who practised mindfulness-based stress reduction therapy for 8 weeks showed clinically meaningful reductions in low back pain and disability that lasted for at least a year, according to findings published in the JAMA (Journal of the American Medical Association).

You can do simple meditation and visualisation techniques at home. According to my clinic experience, the less rules and the easier to do, the more chance it will be done. Using a timer may allow you to relax and not have to mentally keep track of time. Perhaps start with five to ten minutes at first and then extend the duration as you become more practiced.

Committing to do some kind of relaxation and mindfulness practice each day is the goal. Here are my favourite easy meditation options from which you might like to choose:

- **Focus on the breath.** Just sit comfortably with the spine and neck aligned and straight as possible. Preferably close your eyes and just focus on your breathing. No judgement, just observe your breath softly moving in and out. Observe the silence between the breaths. If your mind wanders, no stress, just gently bring it back to focusing on your breath and feel your shoulders, head and jaw relax.

- **Use a mantra.** You may prefer a simple mantra, word or phrase to focus your busy mind. You could use "Om" as your mantra, which has a beautiful low vibrational tone and a long history in Hinduism, Buddhism, meditation and yoga. You could also use a word important to you such as "peace" or "love" or a simple phrase like "just be". Breathing deeply, either vocalise your word or visualise and hear it in your mind.

- **Body relaxation.** Can be done lying down or seated (I prefer to do this lying in bed before sleeping). Close your eyes, take a deep breath and focus and feel your feet. Be aware of the muscles, tendons and ligaments relaxing and softening. Move slowly up the body, gently focusing on each area and feeling it release and relax. Finish with the muscles in the face and around the eyes letting go and then your scalp muscles releasing. Breathe deeply and relax.

- **Positive visualisation.** Get yourself into a comfortable position, close your eyes and take a deep breath. Think about your favourite place to be – your own slice of heaven or your private peaceful place. It might be somewhere you've been in the past or somewhere you would like to go. Imagine it in as much detail as you can and feel yourself there. See yourself as your ideal, perfect self – pain free, moving easily with energy and joy. You are happy, relaxed and grateful for all the blessings in your life. Relax your body, keep breathing deeply and visualise yourself in your perfect place. Really feel yourself there and engage the senses. Can you feel the sunshine? How vibrant are the colours? What can you hear and how does it smell? Smile and imagine yourself enjoying the activities that you do there freely and easily. If you wish, you can even visualise your perfect self, resting and meditating in your peaceful place.

- **Anchor visualisation.** If your mind seems so busy and full and it's hard to focus on only your breath, you might like to use an anchor, an image that gives you strength and stability. For example, you might visualise yourself sitting at the base of a massive tree, strongly rooted into the ground with a huge trunk reaching up into a beautiful blue sky. Or you may see yourself standing and hugging a tree which remains strong even when things are frantic and swirling around.

Spending time and effort on developing a positive attitude, training a strong mind and body are good pain relief strategies. Besides what we have already discussed in this book, other things you might like to try:

- Diversion – rather than being centred on yourself, reaching out to others either for company or to help someone less fortunate than yourself can be rewarding. Even just leaving the house to be amongst people, action and noise can stop being focused on pain.

- Chewing gum can help direct nervous energy.

- Doing something productive with your hands and mind such as crafts or crosswords and puzzles can help the brain switch focus and stop reinforcing pain pathways.

- A good night's sleep is important to help your body heal and for you to cope with pain during the day. Some tips to help you sleep better:

  - Use a comfortable eye mask or blackout curtains to ensure the room is as dark as possible. This helps the body produce melatonin important for a good night's sleep.

  - Go to bed before 10 pm or preferably earlier at the first signs of tiredness. Delaying going to bed when you first feel like it may disrupt your normal sleep cycle. Working with your natural cycle is usually more effective for a good night's sleep.

- Get your daily dose of morning sunshine whenever possible to help produce serotonin – your brain's 'feel good' chemical.

- Magnesium supplements may also help with sleep (and any constipation issues).

- Don't eat before bed. Digestion then becomes a body priority which diverts extra blood supply from your brain to your stomach which can produce interrupted sleep or bad dreams. Ensure that you eat a couple of hours before you retire so that digestion is mostly complete.

- If you snore badly your therapist may be able to help with any jaw or TMJ issues that could be contributing. Alternatively you may need to see your doctor about doing a sleep study.

- Avoid caffeine drinks or stimulants before bed.

Waltz With the Breath

Deep breathing is important to help de-stress the body. A body struggling with shallow breathing and decreased oxygen levels will tend to become acidic and easily trigger the sympathetic nervous system (fight or flight) which can aggravate pain. Slow, diaphragmatic breathing helps the body switch to the parasympathetic nervous system (rest and digest) and stop the production of cortisol, the stress hormone.

If you have been in pain and shallow breathing for a while, it may be difficult to take deep breaths or hold your breath for long periods. Shallow breathing can become habitual or sometimes tight muscles in the back and chest can help create the condition. Bowen Therapy can help to release those muscles and may normalise breathing.

'Waltz with the breath' is a simple, easy three-count technique which is great for beginners. Visit *www.DrugFreePainReliefBook.com* if you'd like to watch the FREE demonstration video.

1. Breathe in through the nose and deeply into the diaphragm for a slow count of three.

2. Hold that breath deep in the lungs for a further count of three.

3. Breathe out through the nose (or pursed lips) to a count of three, then repeat the sequence.

The sequence (slowly):

In, 2, 3

Hold, 2, 3

Out, 2, 3

Repeat three to seven times, then breathe normally.

But sometimes life gets so chaotic and frantic that even when you try the above meditation and breathing techniques, you still can't find those moments of calm and peace. I have two extra strategies for you that may help in those moments:

1. Thought Field Therapy (TFT) – a sequential tapping technique developed by Dr Roger Callahan, a leading American clinical research psychologist, which balances the body's energy system using meridians, or energy pathways, and helps eliminate negative emotions or fears. TFT is safe, non-invasive and unlike other forms of cognitive therapy, the client does not have to relive trauma or talk about details. Having completed TFT training, I find it a useful technique personally and in clinic. To view a BONUS pain relief TFT demonstration, please visit: *www.DrugFreePainReliefBook.com.*

2. Physical and emotional stress release with body therapies. Have you heard that stress and trauma can be held or locked in the body? That can be the negative aspect of 'muscle memory'. Releasing muscles and parts of the body that have held onto a previous trauma can provide emotional relief and restore balance. Once physical and/or

emotional stress has been reduced, it is usually easier to think more clearly and deal with pain. Bowen Therapy gently works with the body to relieve stress and trauma rather than using force. Reflexology, massage and other therapies can also be very useful.

> *"Whatever you do, don't give up!*
> *Commitment, mental toughness and*
> *resilience are key to living a pain free life!"*
>
> **Suzanne McTier-Browne**

My aim has been to provide you with a selection of practical tools to assist you in resolving your pain. There are some other free, practical techniques that may also assist with strengthening your focus and resilience.

Pain Relief Affirmations

Affirmations can be useful to focus on what you really want to achieve and provide a daily reminder to keep you centred on the pathway to pain relief. Affirmations help to counteract negative thought patterns and then retrain, develop and reinforce positive neural pathways.

For many people, lucky numbers are three and seven. Repeating anything a minimum of three times begins to register in the brain. If I'm short for time, I commit to saying my affirmations for the day at least three times, but the ideal would be seven or more.

First thing in the morning and last thing before bed at night, write your affirmations down in a notebook. Then read them out aloud because involving as many of your senses as possible increases success. Writing affirmations in your own handwriting and using different coloured pens also helps with stimulus and impact on the brain. Here are some I use but of course you can also personalise your own:

✓ I am getting stronger and healthier every day and I enjoy life pain free!

✓ I am positive, focused and get good results easily! Life supports me and has my back!

✓ It is safe to let go, I easily release my pain and my past!

✓ Every day I can do more, my life is improving quickly and in perfect ways!

✓ I have a strong back, a good heart and a healthy body that allows me to do what I want to do, life is wonderful!

✓ My mind is focused, my heart is strong and my body is healthy and moves freely!

✓ Life is a blessing and supports me, I can relax and easily release my pain!

✓ I am a warrior with great health, a strong body and a life full of passion!

✓ It is easy for me to move, do my favourite things and enjoy life!

✓ I am relaxed and I move freely with energy and joy. Life is easy for me!

✓ I am happy and healthy, life protects me and keeps me safe!

✓ I am a positive person who makes great decisions and takes action easily!

✓ My mind is strong and my body heals itself in wonderful ways!

✓ Life loves and accepts me, I deserve a good life and a healthy body!

You can also strengthen your affirmations by adding mirror work. In front of a mirror, read or say the affirmation to yourself. Look deep into your own eyes and really commit to the statement you're saying out aloud (minimum three times). Done daily this can become very powerful.

> *"Beliefs have the power to create and the power to destroy. Human beings have the awesome ability to take any experience of their lives and create a meaning that disempowers them or one that can literally save their lives."*
>
> **Tony Robbins**

Now let's go all out! Let's really power up and totally commit. Find happy photos of yourself from a time when you were healthy and without pain (or pictures of what you want to achieve) and display them in prominent places around your bedroom, bathroom and house. Have those ideal images really obvious in your environment, constantly reminding you of your goal.

Whenever you see those images, smile and say to yourself a 'thank you' statement. For example, "Thank you for my wonderful body" or "Thank you for my strong body and moving pain free". Say it sincerely and take a few seconds to imagine that you already have it in your life.

> *"You may feel at times that your body has let you down but strengthening and mastering your mind will guide you to the pain relief and freedom you desire."*
>
> **Suzanne McTier-Browne**

Ultimately we all are part of nature which operates with regular cycles. There are the energetic, busy, growing times that you get in spring and summer when there is lots of sunshine and the days are longer. Then there are the less frantic, rest and recovery times when the days are shorter and it gets colder as in autumn and winter.

Even though we sometimes think mankind is above or separate to the elements, we are still part of that natural cycle. So in your pain relief journey you may well experience periods of activity and progress which are then followed by periods of slow down and enforced rest that weren't necessarily of your choosing. Sometimes things move more slowly than you would like but when life takes over you just have to relax and go with the flow. Controlling stress and remaining positive is a big part of leading a pain free life.

> *"To enjoy good health, to bring true happiness to one's family, to bring peace to all, one must first discipline and control one's own mind."*
>
> **Buddha**

CHAPTER 9

Be the Victor Not the Victim!

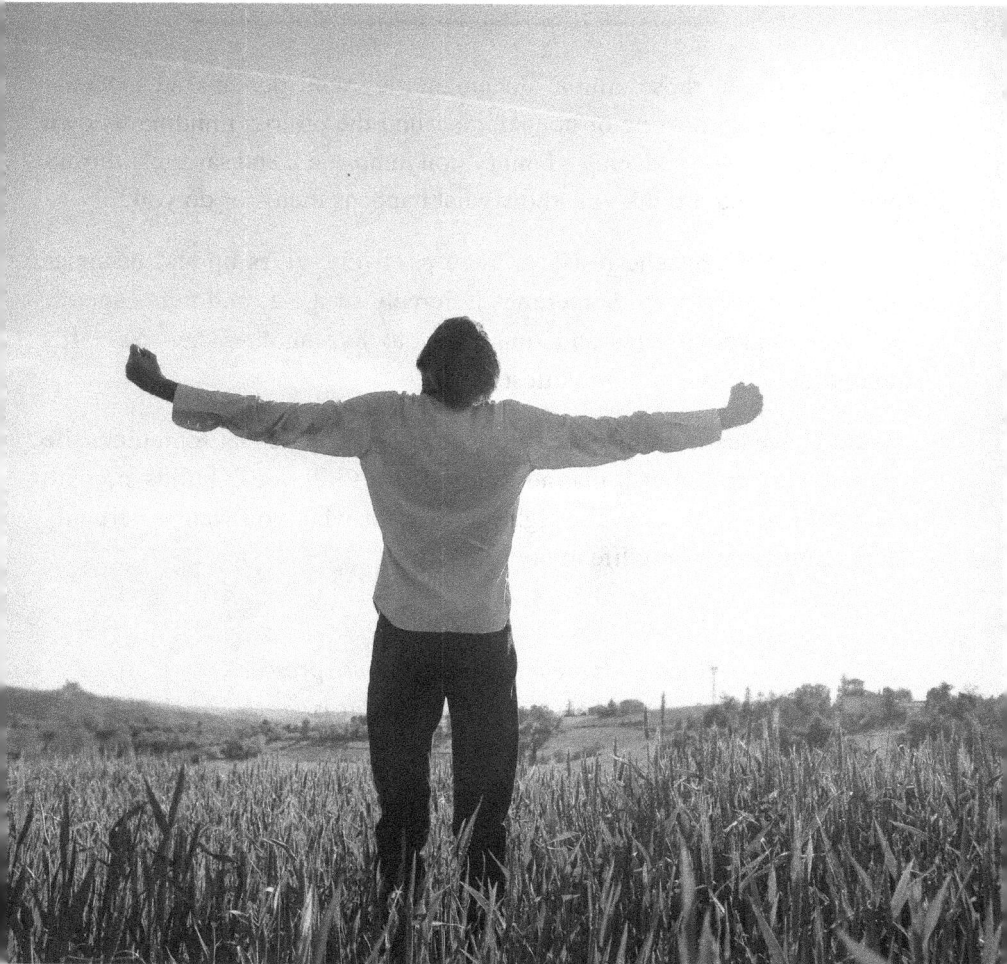

CHAPTER 9

Be the Victor Not the Victim!

> *"Life events, your response, choices and lifestyle have created the body and pain you have today. If you want your body to change and become pain free then you have to change."*
>
> **Suzanne McTier-Browne**

Have you seen those animal documentaries with perhaps an innocent gazelle happily grazing or bouncing around the prairie, minding its own business and then suddenly a hungry lion jumps on it and savagely throws it to the ground. I think you know what happens then – or do you?

Sometimes the gazelle just lays there passively, gives up and becomes dinner without a peep. Sometimes it fiercely struggles and fights against all odds and then wins and runs away to live another day! Yay! It's evolution – 'survival of the fittest'.

What I have learnt from those nature documentaries is that sometimes life can be very cruel but if that adversity doesn't kill you it builds strength and endurance. You have to fight fiercely for what you want – certainly that attitude saved my life many years ago.

> *"Diamonds are made under intense pressure, anything of value, a pain free life is worth fighting for!"*
>
> **Suzanne McTier-Browne**

So Here's the Truth:

If you want to be victorious and beat your pain, you have to also be honest about how you may have contributed. I'm not talking about the original trauma but about what you have done (or not done) since then.

- If you have abused your body for years, don't expect one session with your doctor or therapist to miraculously turn everything around (although sometimes it does). Typically the longer you have had your health issues, the more sessions and effort it takes to address.

- If you are carrying excess weight (particularly around the stomach) realise that structurally it makes you weaker and more prone to accident and re-injury. Step up and take measures to protect yourself.

- No matter how good your doctor or therapist, you are responsible for your actions at home and work. If you are told not to do certain activities but you still continue to do so, then realise that you are risking your recovery and ultimately only hurting yourself. If you persist with old habits that do not serve you then take responsibility and recognise your self-sabotage. That awareness then gives you choice and allows you to make the decision to change.

Are you resisting recovery? Do you really want to get better? Maybe deep down, are you using your pain as an excuse? Maybe it gives you something to talk about and you don't want to let that go? Maybe your pain gets you attention and support from others when you wouldn't normally?

That can be a dangerous game to play. Sometimes your condition can progress so far that it becomes virtually impossible to turn around. So can you get that attention you crave in a more positive way that doesn't jeopardise your health? Perhaps when you become pain free, could you support and help others?

Realise what you have been doing up to this point in your life has helped create your body and perhaps your current pain. Yes there may have been trauma along the way over which you had no control. And if that is the case, I'm so sorry that you've had that experience.

Yes, you may have been dealt a really bad hand in the card game of life. But regardless of what has happened in the past, you have power NOW. You have choice NOW.

If you continue doing what you have always done, then chances are you will continue to get the same results. If you are negative in your outlook, about how you view your body and your future, chances are you will get what you expect – your pain continuing and your health speeding down a negative downward spiral.

Change is key! You are the key! You have more control than you know. In 'Meditation and Yoga Better For Low Back Pain Than Usual Care', Michael Woodhead reports that Curtin University Professor, Peter O'Sullivan, while researching chronic lower back pain found "growing evidence that self-management approaches to manage pain are more effective than usual care, which often focus more on symptom reduction".

The Biology of Belief reviews research in epigenetics and the impact a person's thoughts, perception and subconscious has on their body's healing and aging. Your thoughts and emotions can influence your state of pain and well-being. Dr Lipton has some good news:

> *Your genes do not dictate your life and you can change your life when you change your beliefs ... just eight hours of mindful meditation was sufficient to significantly change vital gene functions ... mindfulness practice can lead to health improvement through profound epigenetic alterations of the genome.*

Let's revisit some Golden Health Rules for pain relief:

- Correcting structural alignment is key to living pain free. Quality bodywork is your best investment.

- Maintaining good posture helps your body work more effectively.

- Be conscious and careful about how you sit, stand and do your everyday activities. Be mindful and move with focus and attention.

- Become your own 'Body Detective' and detect threats in your environment that trigger your pain. Avoid or work safely around those triggers. Don't keep doing activities that cause you pain.

- Regular physical activity helps build and maintain muscle tone, improves circulation, helps decrease stress which will help you increase or maintain mobility and reduce pain levels.

- Exercise doesn't have to be hard, find fun activities that you'll maintain and start slowly and gently.

- Daily stretching is also important. You have to stretch and dissolve that fuzz!

- Drink quality water. The body corrects and muscles release more quickly if you are hydrated. Alcohol, soft drinks (including diet) and coffee tend to dehydrate the body and can deplete valuable vitamins and minerals.

- Eating fresh healthy food is a relatively easy thing you can do to help decrease pain levels. Processed food generally doesn't supply the enzymes, fibre and nutrients for healing and proper body function. Fresh vegetables, fruit and good quality protein are important.

- What you put in your mouth has a huge effect on your pain levels. You might decide to:

  · Decrease the 'white death' in your life – reduce food and drinks high in sugar or containing artificial sweeteners.

  · Support your health with quality, food based vitamin and mineral supplements.

- Depending on your prescribed medications, you might be incorporating vitamin C & D, magnesium, turmeric or ginger into your diet.

- Examine your home and work environment for toxins that could be aggravating your pain, the **4 Ps – People** and **Pollution** (**Places** and **Personal**).

- Practice deep, diaphragmatic breathing and get good sleep.

- Focus and strengthen your mind with tools such as meditation, positive visualisations, TFT and hypnosis.

- Quality bodywork can also help with emotional pain and stress.

- Realise that you have choices. You have the power to choose either negative or positive thoughts. What you think about regularly becomes bigger and your focus in life so choose carefully.

- Repeated thought processes or physical responses, easily become habitual, neural pathways get strengthened and reinforced. If you want your pain to change, you have to change what you have been doing and thinking. Build new pathways, seriously!

- Don't keep doing the same things that haven't helped, you'll just end up strengthening the pain response. Stop doing things that do not serve you!

- You are not alone. It is a sign of intelligence and strength to reach out and get help if you need it. See your doctor or therapist. Additional resources are also listed at the back of this book.

> *"Your health is your most important asset. Invest your time and effort, treat yourself as a priority."*
>
> **Suzanne McTier-Browne**

Beware of Labels!

Some people are so keen to get a diagnosis, they then happily adopt and fully identify with that label. You've probably come across them, they proudly tell everyone their story and how bad they are. It seems no one can help them and they secretly take pride in that.

They may also get rewarded for that pain and diagnosis. Besides attention and sympathy, they might get financial support and assistance that they would not have normally got from the government, family or friends. So a vested interest begins to develop in keeping that pain or condition.

This may be someone you know, or is it you? Perhaps a better strategy is to think of the label as temporary and not focus on it at all. When you decide to fight back, here are some things to consider:

- There's always choice. Choice to fight that label and pain, or not. Choice to give up and do nothing, or to fight back with hope and action. No matter what happens we all have to decide how we respond.

- Remember wherever the mind goes, the body soon follows. A negative mindset usually becomes a self-fulfilling prophecy. There are no medals for being the best example of a worst-case scenario.

- Expectations count! Don't expect one or an occasional episode of pain to be repeated or long lasting. Some people talk themselves into pain. In clinic I sometimes hear negative statements like "I'm always in pain," "It will never go away," "I will never get better," or "My mother had it so I'm sure to". The way you talk to yourself and about yourself is important – stop expecting the worst!

- Just because an authority figure tells you something doesn't mean that they are necessarily right. It may be an opinion or an educated guess. Why do you think people say it is wise to get a second opinion? Or a third opinion? You also don't have to agree. Sometimes you need to just sit quietly for a moment, dig deep inside and see what feels right or resonates for you.

- You have to do more than just talk about getting better. You actually have to get up, take some action and make changes. It takes effort, commitment and a lot of hard work. Big deal! Do it anyway!

- Complaining definitely won't get you better. Moaning and groaning about what a poor life you have doesn't help you or those around you.

- Ultimately it also doesn't matter if someone did wrong and now you are having to deal with the consequences of their action. You are not responsible for your trauma but you are responsible for how you respond.

- Don't compare. It doesn't matter that someone seemingly has had an easier or better life than you. You have to work with the hand that the game of life has given you.

- Don't let lazy mental habits dictate how you feel today. Put effort into starting your day with positive intent, it increases your chances of having a great day!

Are you ready for a boat analogy? You are the captain of your ship. You could have the best crew working for you (the best doctor, therapists and family) doing everything right but if you are a lazy, uncommitted, irresponsible captain, then you could sink that ship at any time (and hurt other people in the process). It all rests with you. The ship sails or sinks depending on your effort and attitude.

How awesome is that? And you thought you were powerless. You are the most important person in this whole process. You have the choice and the power!

> *"Whether you think you can or whether you think you can't, you're right."*
>
> **Henry Ford**

Life disclaimer: now sometimes even when you do everything right, you're in a happy place, not hurting anyone and then life hits you with the proverbial bus (happened to me several times – hate that bus!).

Sometimes life is totally devastating, unfair and no matter what you do you can't turn things around. Sometimes really bad things happen. It shouldn't to good people but it does. Ultimately we have to let it go in some way or it destroys us. All we can do, is do the best with what we have and realise that everyone else is just doing the same.

Case Study – Miracle Ankle

Early in my Bowen Therapy career a massively obese lady came to see me about her chronically painful ankle. She had to book a maxi-taxi to visit the clinic as she couldn't get into her own small car. After her Bowen session, I did not expect huge improvement as ankles (and knees) are weight-bearing joints and therefore can be greatly affected by extra body weight. Once off the table and to the surprise of us both, she started walking immediately without a limp. She had no pain at all and full use of her ankle. I was so happy for her and she rebooked for one more follow-up visit to consolidate the results.

Two days later however, she rang to say that she was cancelling the appointment and was going to see her doctor. I was concerned for her – was she in pain again with her ankle? Her answer was "No" – amazingly it had held the improvement. Her ankle after two years of constant pain and stiffness was now better, but surprisingly she was not happy. She said she didn't know why this had happened and so needed to talk to her doctor. It was hard to understand her anguish when her ankle was physically better and so quickly, surely that was a cause for celebration?

She then told me that she worked from home and that if her ankle was better, she would be expected to go out to pick up and deliver the work. Also, since she had become housebound, friends dropped in frequently to see her, they delivered her groceries, did her errands and paid her bills. Her ankle being better took away her excuse and was going to create massive change in her life.

So some people get fearful and even self-sabotage when pain goes away and their body improves. Some have 'accidents' to get back to where they were originally. They may subconsciously be hiding behind their condition and are sometimes shocked and surprised when they get better so quickly – all of a sudden they have no excuses.

Stop Rehearsing Your Trauma!

In clinic I've noticed a common theme for some in chronic pain. Generally people who respond and heal quickly tend to be those who give me quick and concise details about their medical history just once (with no drama) and then we move on with their recovery.

Others repeatedly tell their story. They might tell my receptionist and other people in the waiting area. They will mention several times during their session and describe in detail their trauma, how excruciating their pain was and continues to be. So in one visit, I may have heard them repeat their story – rehearse their trauma four or five times! And I have to say, that is not for my benefit. You tell me once, I get it.

They are rehearsing their story out aloud because they have now identified so strongly with their condition and they think about it continually, maybe out of habit but also for sympathy and attention. This is ultimately self-defeating behaviour. Living in the past and repeating old history is not doing you good now unless it is your plan to stay that way.

> *"Rehearsing your trauma and repeated negative thinking is like taking poison, it slowly kills your soul and your future. Forgiving yourself and things beyond your control finds freedom!"*
>
> **Suzanne McTier-Browne**

In writing this book, I initially hesitated to talk about my earlier experience with MS because I didn't want to rehearse my own trauma and I only do it now because hopefully it serves a higher purpose in that it might help or empower others.

When I was 22 and fighting my battle, I decided not tell anyone. I didn't tell work colleagues (except my boss), many relatives or friends. Intuitively I realised that I wasn't helping myself by repeating depressing details and I didn't want sympathy or people reminding me how bad things were. It was only many years later after starting the Good Health & Pain Relief Clinic, that I realised my experiences could be useful and may provide hope to others in pain.

That attitude (or stubbornness) of refusing to focus on the diagnosis I think helped save my life. And in hindsight, my pain ended up being a great gift. It made me stand up for myself and fight. It taught me to take responsibility for my own health, to research and ask questions. It ultimately made me stronger, more determined and gave me an ability to help others.

So can I guarantee that if you undertake suggestions in this book that you will live pain free forever – I wish! Of course no one can give you guarantees – life just does not work like that.

> *"Don't be scared of trying something and failing, usually that's the only way to ultimately succeed."*
>
> **Suzanne McTier-Browne**

All you can do is love yourself enough to do your very best. Invest in your health and support yourself with a great team of honest and talented people who have your best interests at heart. Be grateful for the good things already in your life. Really appreciate the people who love you and enjoy wholeheartedly the moments of happiness and beauty that the universe gives you. Love and best wishes!

CHAPTER 10

Support at Home

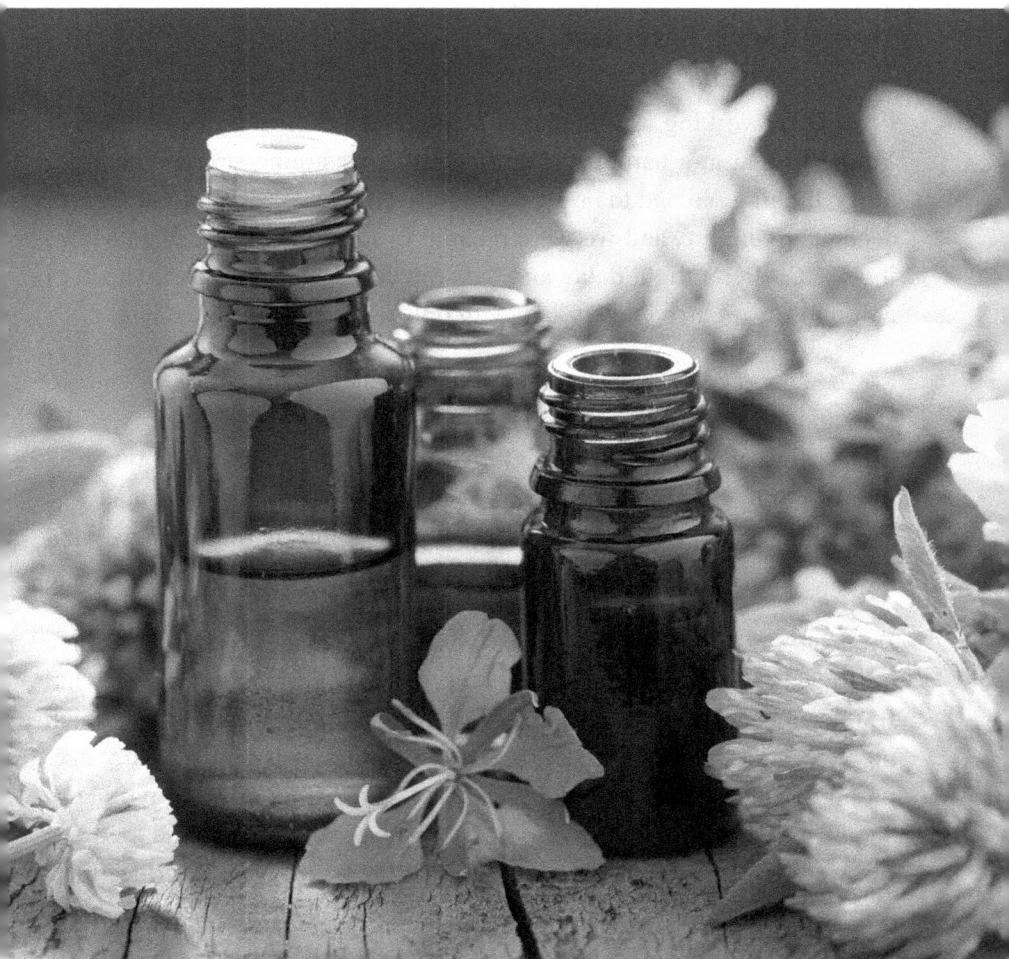

Support at Home

Not all of us live in a capital city or area rich in therapists and other resources. Sometimes you've got to put effort into getting yourself organised at home in order to help yourself. Following are a couple of my favourite things that may assist and support you.

Young Living Essential Oils

I had been working as a therapist for several years when I came across Young Living at a natural therapies expo. I was quite stressed and in a hurry, nothing seemed to be going right that day. My husband, Steve, was accompanying me, and we were rushing to see things at the expo before it closed. After a flight delay and then the taxi driver from hell who kept getting lost, we arrived very late with only an hour or so to closing.

Steve had wrenched his back during the trip and I didn't have the time to stop and help him as we rushed around. I felt sorry for him, angry at the flight delay, the incompetent taxi driver and worried about the time. So when I got to the Young Living stall half an hour before closing and was asked if I wanted to try some essential oils, I honestly didn't know what to say.

I was obviously really tense and so was offered some oils while I lay on a massage table for a minute. **Valor** was applied to the soles of my feet and I inhaled **Peace & Calming**. Quickly I noticed that I was feeling much more relaxed and settled. Poor Steve was waiting patiently by my side but in discomfort from his tight back so I asked if there was anything to soothe and relieve his tense muscles. **Panaway** was applied and then in a rush I got a wholesale account and bought the Everyday Oils collection.

Back at our hotel, it dawned on me what had actually happened. I had gone from being very tense and frazzled to becoming relaxed and calm in a surprisingly short period of time. I asked Steve if he needed help but he said he was fine. That was the start of my love affair with Young Living Essential Oils.

It's about ten years now that I have been using the oils and supplements with my family and in clinic. I have found them invaluable in so many ways. I use the household and body care products to help reduce my family's exposure to harmful chemicals and toxins. When life gets busy it is extra support for when I don't eat perfectly or get enough rest. Some of my particular favourites are: **Ningxia Red, OmegaGize, Longevity, Mineral Essence, BLM, Sulfurzyme, AgilEase, Cool Azul Cream** or **Gel, Panaway, Deep Relief** and **Stress Away**.

I'm often asked how I use Young Living in a typical day, so as a general guide here is what I do:

Morning – Wake Up Routine	Inhale or wear as a perfume **Peppermint** and **Joy** oils. Depending on how I feel, might alternate with **White Angelica, Ylang Ylang, Valor, Awaken or Motivation**.
	Apply **Endoflex** to my throat area and **Progressence Phyto Plus** on my wrists to help keep me happy and balanced.
	In the bathroom, I have **Thieves Foaming Hand Soap** to wash my hands and face. I either clean my teeth with **Thieves Ultra Toothpaste** (or **Aromabright** if I feel my teeth need some brightening) or gargle with **Thieves Mouthwash.**
	I have my **Meadow Mist Aroma Guard Deodorant** but if I'm travelling and want to reduce luggage, I'll often use a light smear of my **Thieves Hand Sanitiser** to keep me fresh.
	I also love a cup of warm water with a drop of **Lemon** oil first thing in the morning. Fresh lemon juice is also good but I found I was getting sore gums so since then I've switched to **Lemon** essential oil and there's been no problem.

Before and After Exercise	One drop of **Peppermint** oil in my water bottle helps me wake up and keep invigorated. If I'm tired and not wanting to exercise, a dose of **Ningxia Red** before my session or in my water bottle also helps me commit to a great workout.
	If my muscles are tight from work or exercising, I apply **Aroma Siez**, **Wintergreen** or **Peppermint** to the affected area or use my **Deep Relief Roll-on**. **Cool Azul Sports Gel** is also easy to use.
	After an exercise session, I freshen up and shower with **Morning Start Bath & Shower Gel**.
Breakfast	I love eggs or protein for breakfast but if I have a busy day and can't sit down to eat, I'll make a healthy smoothie. My favourite ingredients to work with are:
	• Organic baby spinach
	• Organic banana or blueberries
	• Quality vitamin C powder with bioflavonoids
	• Magnesium powder
	• **Balance Complete** or **Power Meal**
	• **Mineral Essence**
	• **Ningxia Red**
	• Turmeric and ginger raw and grated (or organic powder)
	• Cold filtered water and ice
	• Spritz it all up in a blender, pour into a travel mug and you are ready to go!
Daily Supplements	If I've had my smoothie for breakfast (as above), I might additionally take:
	OmegaGize (so convenient, three supplements in one – Omega-3 fatty acids, CoQ10 (ubiquinone) and Vitamin D-3)
	Longevity
	BLM, Sulfurzyme or **AgilEase** (if I'm feeling a bit stiff and want some extra support for my muscles and joints)

At Work	I have to keep mentally alert and focused so I'll often inhale or wear as a perfume any of the following: **Clarity, Brain Power, En-r-gee, Valor, Peppermint, Magnify My Purpose, Build Your Dream, Believe, Highest Potential or Cedarwood.**
	I diffuse oils in my clinic and everyone enjoys coming to such a relaxed and peaceful space. I choose what oils I diffuse depending on the clients I'll be seeing. For new clients, I may use **Joy** and **Peace & Calming** to help calm and reassure. If it's winter, I'll diffuse **Thieves** or **Purification** to maintain and support a healthy environment.
	To relax clients with tight muscles before I see them, I may offer **Release, Aroma Siez, Panaway, Deep Relief** or **Stress Away. Ortho Sport or Ease** are favourite massage oils.
	For busy and stressed clients, **Peace & Calming, Stress Away, Sacred Mountain, White Angelica** and **Release** can be useful.
	Later in the afternoon of a busy day, I may have a second dose of **Ningxia Red** with a drop of **Peppermint** to help maintain focus and energy.
Evening Before Bed	I like to use products that are free of harmful chemicals so I take my make-up off with either **Orange Blossom Facial Wash** or the **ART Gentle Cleanser.** Twice a week I love using the **Satin Facial Scrub** to gently exfoliate.
	I shower with **Evening Peace Bath & Shower Gel** and wash my hair with **Lavender** or **Copaiba Vanilla Moisturising Shampoo** and **Conditioner.** It's great to know I'm not washing in toxic chemicals.
	I apply **Frankincense** to my face and then over the top either **ART Light Moisturizer** or **Boswellia Wrinkle Cream** (my favourite for winter). Alternatively I might use a drop of **Lavender** and **Geranium** mixed with a teaspoon of organic coconut oil to moisturise my face, neck and chest.
	If I'm feeling some tightness after a long day, I might apply **Deep Relief** or **Stress Away Roll-on, Aroma Siez** or **Cool Azul Sports Gel.**
	If stressed, I'll inhale or wear before I go to bed – **Lavender, Stress Away, Peace & Calming, Dream Catcher, Forgiveness, Gratitude, Hope, Joy, Release, RutaVaLa, Sacred Mountain, Surrender or White Angelica.** My bedside table is crammed with essential oils!

Please note: Any information regarding essential oils are for general adult use only and Young Living Therapeutic Grade Essential Oils, that is the only brand I use and trust.

Do It Yourself

If you are feeling stiff or have tight muscles plus you like DIY, you can also personalise your own relaxing comfort oil to rub on those stressed areas. For example, I love mixing ten drops of **Release** with ten drops of either **Stress Away, Valor, Wintergreen, Marjoram, Rosemary** or **Peppermint** (just select your favourite or you can choose a different oil). Mix into quarter of a cup of cold pressed unrefined coconut oil. You only use a small amount at a time and kept in a small sealed container, your personalised mix will last for many applications. **Lavender** and **Copaiba** is also a soothing combination.

Another DIY option is to make up your own simple **Body Soak**:

375 g packet of Epsom Salts

1/2 cup of fine Himalayan Salt or Dead Sea Salt

10 – 15 drops of your favourite essential oils

(you might like to try **Aroma Siez, Relieve It** or any of the oils mentioned previously)

Combine thoroughly and place in an air-tight container. Depending on the size of you and your bath, this would typically do two baths for a small adult (or around five foot or hand soaks). Get into a warm bath with your personalised body soak and relax for 10–20 minutes. Get out of the bath while the water is still warm, gently towel dry but do not rinse. Jump straight into bed and have a good night's sleep!

If you have any questions or would like to access Young Living products, please contact the person who introduced you (details are listed in Recommended Resources at the back of this book). If no-one introduced you, please visit: *www.yldist.com/suzannemctierbrowne.*

The Power in You!

I intuitively understood early in my own journey and battle with pain, how important it was to develop a strong mind and resilience. Research now confirms this, in *The Biology of Belief*, Dr Lipton writes:

> *The primary source controlling our life experiences is the subconscious mind, and we need to focus on re-programming it rather than just shifting our conscious mind's beliefs...belief exerts a powerful influence over physiology, gene expression, and behaviour.*

So controlling negative thought patterns and emotional responses to pain and stress may hold the key to success and achieving pain relief. There is a powerful force inside everyone that, once unlocked, can make any dream, vision, or desire become a reality.

You have the potential to have a life filled with more passion, confidence, joy and love than you ever dreamed possible. Science has now confirmed what hypnotherapists have always believed. Hypnosis is not just in the mind, but rather it is the means of connecting the body and the mind together. Hypnosis can be a valuable tool, and one that you can now access at home.

Self-Hypnosis to Transform Your Life

Someone I greatly respect, a master hypnotist with more than 25 years' experience is Darren Stephens. Recognised as one of the World's Fastest Hypnotists, Darren has developed a breakthrough range of tools to help people achieve their goals and live the life they were born to live. Your mindset is the key to your success.

Darren's **Pain Control Hypnosis Collection** was designed to help you battle pain. Whether you are healing after an operation or injury, or you are dealing with chronic illness or disability, or even if you just have a headache, the techniques contained in this program will help you take back control.

See the Recommended Resources section at the back of this book for more information.

About the Author

Suzanne McTier-Browne

Author & Therapist

Suzanne is an author, a certified Advanced Bowen Therapist, Reflexologist and Massage Therapist.

At the age of 22, Suzanne was diagnosed with multiple sclerosis. At the time, there were no treatments for the life-threatening disease. In pain and given just 12 months to live, she began her own investigations into the condition. Thanks to her personal initiative and specific natural therapies, she overcame MS.

Just one year later she contracted Ross River Fever which she also overcame through personal research and natural therapies. Having survived illnesses in her own life, her mission now is to empower and support people in their health and wellness.

After a successful 19-year career in business management, Suzanne decided to start her own business in natural therapies. Through her Good Health & Pain Relief Clinic in Rockhampton, Queensland, Australia, Suzanne has been able to empower more than 2,000 clients to relieve their pain.

In addition to her training and more than 17 years of experience as a therapist, Suzanne holds a bachelor's degree in arts where she majored in journalism, Japanese, and communications. She also holds a graduate diploma in management and a master's degree in business administration.

During her career in business management and as a therapist, Suzanne has worked with many organisations including ANZ Banking Group, Ansett Resort & Hotels (Hayman Island), Central Queensland University, The Family Medical Practice at Kmart Plaza and The Glenmore Family Medical Practice.

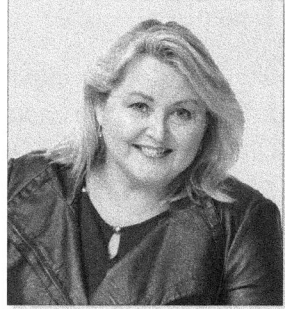

Suzanne's professional associations include The Bowen Association of Australia, The Reflexology Association of Australia, and Massage & Myotherapy Australia (previously the Australian Association of Massage Therapists).

She has worked internationally and travelled throughout Japan, Hong Kong, Korea, Singapore, China, Fiji, Vanuatu, Vila, Cook Islands, the United States, Ecuador, Puerto Rico, the Caribbean, Greece, Italy, France, Germany, Switzerland, Austria, Denmark, Turkey, Croatia and the United Kingdom.

Suzanne McTier-Browne is the author of Drug Free Pain Relief and lives in Queensland, Australia.

RECOMMENDED
RESOURCES

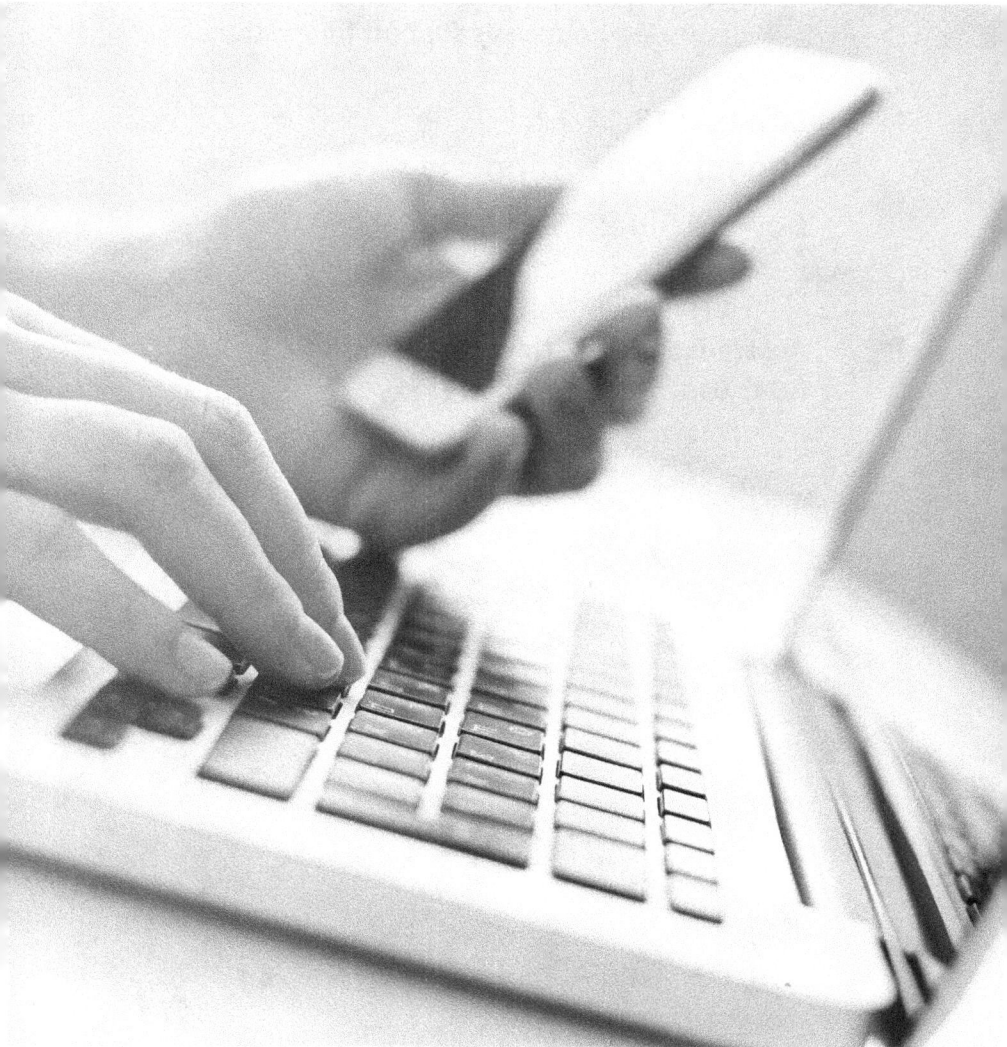

Recommended Resources

Is your pain getting you down?
Need to talk to someone now? Make the call for help.

If you can't get to your doctor,
phone 24-hour crisis support (in Australia):

Lifeline: 13 11 14

1800RESPECT: 1800 737 732

Beyond Blue: 1300 224636

Or in an emergency, phone:

Australia: 000 **New Zealand: 111**
USA: 911 **UK: 999**

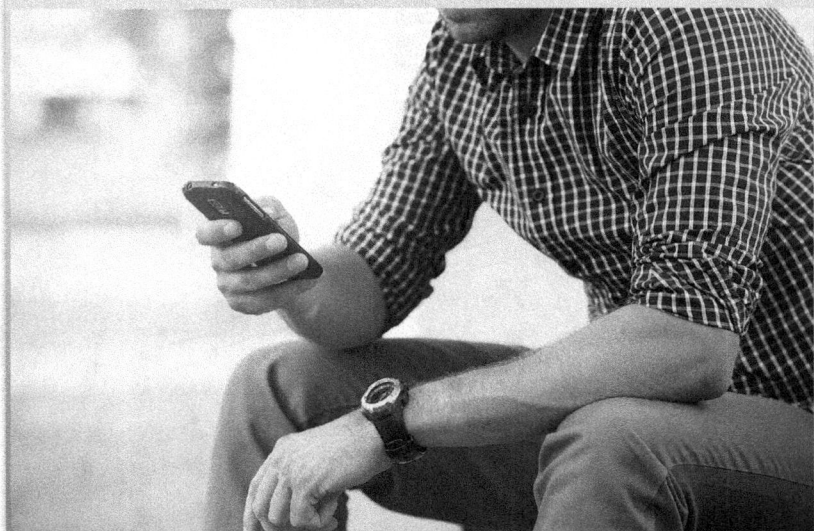

Pain Control Collection

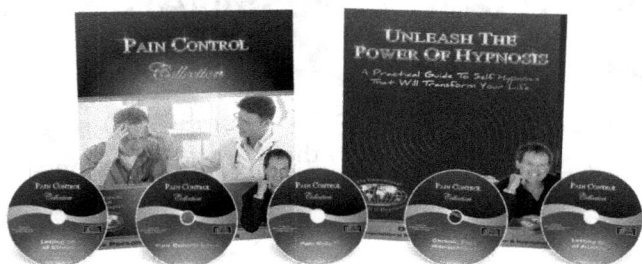

Although pain is an important signal from the body that something needs attention, and no unusual pain should just be ignored, it is useful to remember that the experience of pain always includes a psychological component.

And that means that you can influence the experience of pain.

The **Pain Control Hypnosis Collection** from the *Darren Stephens Personal Enhancement Series* was designed to help you battle pain. Whether you are healing after an operation or injury, or whether you are dealing with chronic illness or disability, or even if you just have a headache, the techniques contained in this program will stand you in good stead.

This collection includes these 5 tracks essential for controlling pain:

- **Letting Go of Stress** is an essential tool which will empower your sense of autonomy and control and allow you to relax and sleep peacefully
- **Your Control Panel** gives you the key to success for, and the ultimate control system to enhance, every function of your mind and body including your pain centres
- **Letting Go of Anxiety** will help to ensure you stay calm in stressful situations and teach you to stop assuming the worst which exacerbates painful symptoms
- **Pain Relief** has been put together specifically to help you modify, dull or remove the experience of pain
- **Chronic Pain Management** will empower anyone suffering from chronic conditions to significantly affect the levels of pain that they encounter

DARREN J STEPHENS
PERSONAL ENHANCEMENT SERIES

http://bit.ly/hypnosis_001

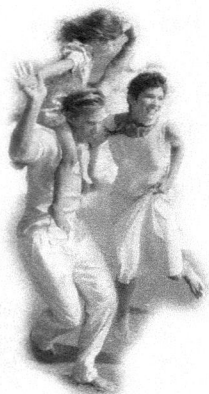

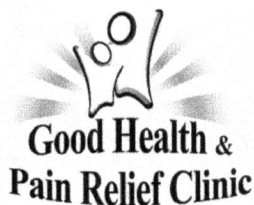

Professional Associations:

Bowen Association of Australia	P: 1300 780 638 E: admin@bowen.org.au
Bowen Therapy Academy of Australia	P: 03 5572 3000 E: bowtech@h140.aone.net.au
Bowen Training Australia	E: info@bowentraining.com.au
Bowen Association UK	P: 01205 319100 E: office@bowen-technique.co.uk
Bowen Training UK	P: 0700 269 3685 E: office@bowentraining.co.uk
BowenUSA	E: ContactUs@BowenUSA.org
American Bowen Academy	P: 866 862 6936 (Toll Free)
Reflexology Assoc of Australia	P: 1300 733 711 E: admin@reflexology.org.au
Baby Reflexology	P: 01865 340320 E: info@babyreflex.co.uk
Massage & Myotherapy Australia	Level 8, 53 Queen Street, Melbourne, P: 1300 138 872 E: info@massagemyotherapy.com.au

Young Living Essential Oils

If you have questions, would like assistance or more information, please contact:

Name: _____

Phone: _____

Email: _____

Member No: _____ *(your sponsor & enroller)*

References / Bibliography

Introduction

Pain Australia, http://www.painaustralia.org.au/advocacy/pa_advocacy.html, accessed 10/10/16.

American Academy of Pain Medicine, http://www.painmed.org/patientcenter/facts-on-pain/, accessed 10/10/16.

Determinants of Increased Opioid-Related Mortality in the United States and Canada, 1990–2013: A Systematic Review, Nicholas B. King, PhD, Veronique Fraser, RN, MSc, Constantina Boikos, MSc, Robin Richardson, MPH, and Sam Harper, PhD, http://ajph.aphapublications.org/doi/full/10.2105/AJPH.2014.301966, accessed 14/4/17.

'800 Australians die per year from prescription drug overdoses, experts say', by Sarah Whyte, http://www.abc.net.au/news/2017-04-13/800-australians-overdose-on-prescription-drugs-per-year-experts/8443578, accessed 14/4/1.

Chapter 1

Lady Cilento on Vitamin and Mineral Deficiencies, 1986, Pitman Publishing Ptd Ltd, South Melbourne pp, 10, 27–30.

The Cilento Way, The Sunday Mail publication, 1984, Queensland Newspapers Pty Ltd, Bowen Hills.

https://www.mssociety.org.uk/what-is-ms/information-about-ms/about-ms, accessed 14/12/16.

Food as Medicine, Earl Mindell, R. Ph, Ph.D., 1994, Fireside New York p.52.

Good Health in the 21st Century, Dr Carole Hungerford, 2009, Scribe Publications Pty Ltd, p.172.

Nourishing Traditions, Sally Fallon with Mary G Enig, Phd, 2001, Revised Second Edition, New Trends Publishing Inc, Washington DC, p.51.

Take Control of Your Health and Escape the Sickness Industry, 11th ed, Elaine Hollingsworth, 2010, Empowerment Press International, Mudgeeraba, p.99.

Chapter 2

http://www.mydr.com.au/pain/pain-and-how-you-sense-it, accessed 29/5/17.

The Bowen Technique, John Wilks, 2007, CYMA Ltd, Dorset, UK, p.91.

http://www.painaustralia.org.au/for-everyone/what-is-pain.html.

http://mydr.com.au/pain/meditation-and-yoga-better-for-low-back-pain-than-usual-care, by Michael Woodhead, accessed 12/2/17.

The Biology of Belief, Bruce H. Lipton, Ph.D, 10th Anniversary Edition, 2015, Hay House Australia Pty Ltd, p.140.

http://www.painaustralia.org.au/advocacy/pa_advocacy.html, accessed 12/2/21017.

Chapter 3

Bowen Unravelled, Julian Baker, 2014, Lotus Publishing, Chichester, p.42.

The Bowen Technique – The Inside Story by John Wilks 2007, CYMA Ltd, Dorset, UK.

Healthy Soul, April 8, 2016, http://www.healthysoul.co.uk/tag/bear-grylls/.

Chapter 4

https://bowenbtpa.wordpress.com/2015/02/10/world-champion-motorbike-racer-james-ellison-claims-bowen-therapy-has-changed-his-life/.

http://www.saga.co.uk/magazine/health-wellbeing/treatments/bowen-technique.aspx, 17/9/13, accessed 14/12/2016.

Total Reflexology, US Edition, Martine Faure-Alderson, 2008, Healing Arts Press, Vermont, pp 2,4.

Reflexology, Inge Dougans, 2005,Thorsons, London, pp 3-6.

Nature & Health Magazine article (Dec 2016 – Jan 2017, p.30).

http://www.doctoroz.com/article/massage-therapy-can-help-these-5-painful-conditions, accessed 14/12/16.

Chapter 5

Dr Gil Hedley, 'The Fuzz Speech' video (https://www.youtube.com/watch?v=BdRqLrCF_Ys,published 18/4/2012).

Chapter 6

Total Reflexology, US Edition, Martine Faure-Alderson, 2008, Healing Arts Press, Vermont. pp 109–112.

Joint Health Magazine, 'How Can Soft Drinks Worsen Your Osteoarthritis and Joint Pain?', https://www.jointhealthmagazine.com/how-can-soft-drinks-worsen-your-osteoarthritis-and-joint-pain.html, Janice Carson, accessed 19/4/17.

Dr Oz TV show October 3, 2014, http://www.doctoroz.com/episode/new-dangers-artificial-sweeteners?video_id=3323249357001.

The Cilento Way, The Sunday Mail publication, 1984, Queensland Newspapers Pty Ltd, Bowen Hills.

Good Health in the 21st Century, Dr Carole Hungerford, 2009, Scribe Publications Pty Ltd, p. 172.

The Vitamin D Solution Australian Edition, 2010, Michael F Holick, Phd, MD, Scribe Publications, Melbourne.

Nourishing Traditions, Sally Fallon with Mary G Enig, Phd, 2001, Revised Second Edition, New Trends Publishing Inc, Washington DC, p.42.

Magnesium – The Miracle Mineral, Dr Sandra Cabot, 2007, WHAS Pty Ltd Camden NSW.

Outsmart Sugar: How to Retrain Your Brain to Kick the Sugar Habit, 2016, Tara C. Mitchell, Global Publishing Group, Mt Evelyn, Victoria, Australia.

Take Control of Your Health and Escape the Sickness Industry, Elaine Hollingsworth, 11th edition, 2010, Empowerment Press International, Mudgeeraba, pp. 312,313.

http://www.webmd.com/osteoarthritis/news/20121108/soda-may-worsen-knee-osteoarthritis-in-men#1 by Charlene Laino, accessed 19/4/17.

Dr Joseph Mercola, (Mercola 2015) (http://articles.mercola.com/sites/articles/archive/2015/09/21/golden-milk.aspx).

Healthy and Natural World 2016 (http://www.healthyandnaturalworld.com/how-to-make-anti-inflammatory-turmeric-ginger-tea.

Modern Ailments Ancient Remedies, Gillian Kerr and Dr Yvonne Bloomfield, 1998, Lansdowne Publishing Pty Ltd, Sydney.

http://www.doctoroz.com/blog/mao-shing-ni-lac-dom-phd/4-herbs-natural-pain-relief.

Chapter 7

The Biology of Belief, Bruce H. Lipton, Ph.D, 10th Anniversary Edition, 2015, Hay House Australia Pty Ltd, p. 162.

Slow Death by Rubber Duck, Rick Smith, Bruce Lourie, 2010, University of Queensland Press, St Lucia.

https://www.betterhealth.vic.gov.au/health/healthyliving/mobile-phones-and-your-health.

http://www.laughteronlineuniversity.com/norman-cousins-a-laughterpain-case-study/.

The Pulse Test: The Secret Of Building Your Basic Health, Arthur F. Coca, 1982, Barricade Books.

"A study of interior landscape plants for indoor air pollution abatement" (Report). BC Wolver ton; WL Douglas; K Bounds (July 1989). NASA. NASA-TM-108061.

How to Grow Fresh Air, BC Wolverton, 1996, New York, Penguin Books.

Chapter 8

The Biology of Belief, Bruce H. Lipton, Ph.D, 10th Anniversary Edition, 2015, Hay House Australia Pty Ltd, pp. 139, 140.

http://www.mydr.com.au/pain/meditation-and-yoga-better-for-low-back-pain-than-usual-care, by Michael Woodhead, accessed 12/2/17.

Chapter 9

http://www.mydr.com.au/pain/meditation-and-yoga-better-for-low-back-pain-than-usual-care, by Michael Woodhead, accessed 12/2/17.

The Biology of Belief, Bruce H. Lipton, Ph.D, 10th Anniversary Edition, 2015, Hay House Australia Pty Ltd, pp. 142, 144, 145 & 147.